Advances and Challenges in Urine Laboratory Analysis

Edited by Tomasz Jarzembowski and Agnieszka Daca

Published in London, United Kingdom

Advances and Challenges in Urine Laboratory Analysis
http://dx.doi.org/10.5772/intechopen.104336
Edited by Tomasz Jarzembowski and Agnieszka Daca

Contributors
Jorge Alberto Cortés, Laura Cristina Nocua-Báez, Kumar Venkitanarayanan, Abraham Joseph Pellissery, Poonam Gopika Vinayamohan, Leya Susan Viju, Divya Jopseph, Hiroko Furo, Sarah Abdelsayed, Tony Lin, Yi Yuan Zhou, Chandrasekhar Nagaraj, Noren Villalobos, Lovelesh K. Kumar Nigam, Agnieszka Daca, Tomas Jarzembowski

First published in London, United Kingdom, 2024 by IntechOpen
IntechOpen is the global imprint of INTECHOPEN LIMITED, registered in England and Wales, registration number: 11086078, 5 Princes Gate Court, London, SW7 2QJ, United Kingdom

British Library Cataloguing-in-Publication Data
A catalogue record for this book is available from the British Library

Additional hard and PDF copies can be obtained from orders@intechopen.com

Advances and Challenges in Urine Laboratory Analysis
Edited by Tomasz Jarzembowski and Agnieszka Daca
p. cm.
Print ISBN 978-1-83768-484-7
Online ISBN 978-1-83768-485-4
eBook (PDF) ISBN 978-1-83768-486-1

For EU product safety concerns:
IN TECH d.o.o., Prolaz Marije Krucifikse Kozulić 3, 51000 Rijeka, Croatia,
info@intechopen.com or visit our website at intechopen.com.

Meet the editors

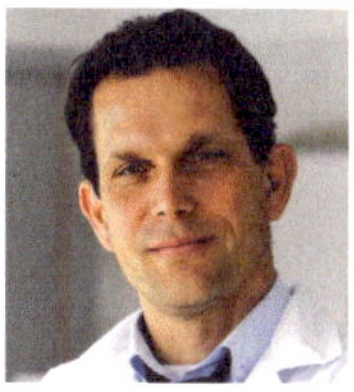

Tomasz Jarzembowski is an assistant professor in the Department of Microbiology, Medical University of Gdańsk (GUMed), Poland. He obtained a Ph.D. from the Department of Biology, University of Gdańsk (UG), in 2000, and a DSc from the Faculty of Medicine, GUMed, in 2015. After obtaining a specialization in clinical microbiology in 2003, Dr. Jarzembowski began studying biofilm formation and heterogeneity of antibiotic resistance. The latter research, which he conducted in cooperation with experts in nephrology and immunology, resulted in the designation of a new diagnostic method for UTIs, which was patented in 2017. Currently, his interests are focused on the proteomic study of virulence biomarkers of species of microbiome. Dr. Jarzembowski has been a leader of several projects of the Ministry of Education and Science, Poland, and a grant from Applied Microbiology International. He is a member of the Main Audit Committee of the Polish Society of Microbiologists (PTM), the Steering Committee of the Gdańsk branch of PTM, Applied Microbiology International, and the editorial board of several international journals. He is an author and editor of more than sixty scientific publications and book chapters.

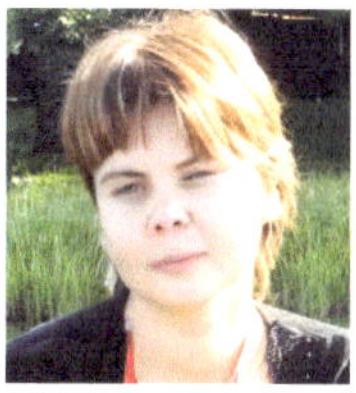

Agnieszka Daca obtained her Ph.D. from the Medical University of Gdańsk, Poland, in 2011. Her thesis discussed immunological changes observed in the blood of patients with systemic lupus erythematosus (SLE). After her Ph.D., Dr. Daca divided her work into two aspects. The first is the widely understood interaction between bacteria and the innate immune system (especially monocytes) in cooperation with Tomasz Jarzembowski. For this, she researches virulence traits of bacteria (especially Enterococcus faecalis) and their impact on monocytes' behavior. The main aspect is the monocytes' ability to phagocytose bacteria and their impact on the human body's ability to eradicate bacteria, especially in immunocompromised patients. The second branch of her scientific activity is the immunology of autoimmune diseases, mainly SLE and antineutrophil cytoplasmic antibody (ANCA)-associated vasculitis in cooperation with Prof. Alicja Dębska-Ślizień and her co-workers from the Medical University of Gdańsk.

Contents

Preface

Urinalysis is one of the most useful laboratory techniques that provides an abundance of information regarding one's health. In most circumstances, it is non-invasive and safe. Aside from its obvious benefits, urinalysis reflects not only urinary tract functioning but also the functioning of other parts of the body such as the digestive system or circulatory system. The various biomarkers and metabolites detected in urine can provide information about ongoing processes and currently developing problems in the body. Given the wide range of possible applications for data received from urine analysis in everyday home and hospital care, it is not unexpected that urinalysis history is particularly long and interesting.

The first glimpse into rudimental urine analysis, known at the time as uroscopy, comes from ancient history. Back then, sages were aware of urine's unique ability to represent the human body condition and were able to link features of urine such as color, consistency, sediment, odor, and volume with, for example, the state of hydration or the diet of the urine donor. The drawn findings became more sophisticated and better reflected the state of homeostasis of the human body as understanding about the functioning of the urinary system in general and each of its parts independently increased.

The advancement of understanding the human body's functioning in health and disease was matched by the development of increasingly precise and accurate diagnostic tools. The data acquired from correctly collected urine is now astounding. However, it is worth noting that the increasing specificity, susceptibility, and diversity of urine analysis techniques corresponds to the growing demand for such procedures. It no longer simply reflects the body's volemia state, it also indicates numerous diseases, pharmacokinetics, and many other factors.

The advancement of renal transplants has created a demand for accurate monitoring of kidney functioning without the use of invasive procedures. The patients' near-constant monitoring necessitates both swift and sensitive approaches for assessing the current state of the transplanted organ as well as the entire body. This includes, for example, normally difficult-to-discover asymptomatic inflammations, which, due to their insidious nature, can lead to transplant rejection.

We cordially welcome you to read this book. It highlights the history of urinalysis and its significance in daily practice as well as in the case of patients with unique needs and requirements. We hope you will find it informative and stimulating.

Agnieszka Daca and Tomasz Jarzembowski
Departamet of Medical Microbiology,
Medical University of Gdańsk,
Gdańsk, Poland

Foreword

Urine was the first body fluid to be examined in order to find associations between its changed properties (looks, odor, and taste) and various human ailments. Urinoscopy, and then urinalysis in its most rudimentary form, was already known more than 6000 years ago. Modern urinalysis started in the 17th century and progress is ongoing. This book provides a comprehensive overview of urinalysis.

Chapter 1 by Dr. Agnieszka Daca and D.Sc. Tomasz Jarzembowski reviews the history of urinalysis and highlights its progress over the years.

Chapter 2 by Prof. Chandrasekhar Nagaraj discusses catheter-associated urinary tract infections (CAUTIs). UTIs are of great clinical importance and often arise as nosocomial infections, originating in the hospital setting. In cases of hospital-acquired UTIs (HAUTIs), patients' hospital stays are often prolonged and costly. Even worse, microorganisms that cause HAUTIs are more virulent and resistant to antibiotics than those causing other UTIs. The ability of such microorganisms to form biofilm on catheters often leads to catheter-associated UTIs (CAUTIs), which are the second most common hospital-acquired infection (HAI). This chapter describes the CAUTI condition itself, as well as procedures preceding catheterization, catheterization itself, and other preventive measures.

Chapter 3 by Dr. Laura Cristina Nocua-Báez and Dr. Jorge Alberto Cortés also reviews UTIs. Apart from obvious microbiological approaches, there are non-microbiological tests for characterizing the microorganisms that cause UTIs. Some of these tests can be used in the doctor's office or emergency room, whereas others require more sophisticated instruments. Some of the goals of using non-microbiological approaches are to bypass the difficulties of diagnosis in some patients (e.g., older patients or those who are cognitively impaired) and to more quickly diagnose UTIs, enabling quicker introduction of therapy.

Chapter 4 by Dr. Lovelesh K. Nigam discusses patients undergoing renal transplants. These patients may develop UTIs, cystitis, nephrolithiasis, cancers, and other conditions that can be traced and diagnosed by modern urinalysis. One of the important groups of conditions for which transplant patients are at risk, and for which urinalysis may help with early detection, is viral nephropathies. Furthermore, modern urinalysis may indicate upcoming graft rejection as well as the condition of the graft itself, reducing the need for renal biopsy and related risks. Finally, urinalysis in this group of patients may show the relapse of the disease underlying kidney failure prior to transplantation.

Chapter 5 by Dr. Abraham Joseph Pellissery, Dr. Poonam Gopika Vinayamohan, Ms. Leya Susan Viju, Ms. Divya Joseph, and Prof. Kumar Venkitanarayanan discuss urine metabolomics. By discovering novel biomarkers, the metabolomics approach helps to develop new avenues of clinical diagnosis not only for diseases of the urinary system, but also for infectious, metabolic, and inflammatory diseases and malignancies. It is also invaluable in monitoring health status, both in healthy and diseased individuals. In the former, it may give early warning, while in the latter it may show the progression of the disease or the progression and efficacy of treatment.

Chapter 6 by Assistant Prof. Hiroko Furo, Dr. Tony Lin, Dr. Yi Yuan Zhou and Dr. Sarah Abdelsayed discusses the application of quantitative gas chromatography–mass spectrometry (GC–MS) for tracing opiates in urine. Findings from GC–MS may help clinicians monitor the results of treatment for opioid use disorder, as well as facilitate interpretation of urine drug test results.

Finally, in Chapter 7, which examines UTIs in pregnant women, Ph.D. Noren Villalobos shows that the use of non-microbiological tests assessing the possibility of UTIs in this vulnerable group of patients may facilitate diagnosis (including the identification of involved microorganisms) and thus allow for proper, timely, and targeted treatment.

In conclusion, modern urinalysis is a relatively easy, multimodal, and fairly inexpensive tool in health and disease monitoring, as excellently described and discussed in this book.

Jacek Witkowski
Professor,
Head of the Department of Physiopathology,
Faculty of Medicine,
Medical University of Gdańsk,
Gdańsk, Poland

Section 1

Urinalysis in Everyday Practice

Chapter 1

Introductory Chapter: Modern Diagnostics with the Ancient History

Agnieszka Daca and Tomasz Jarzembowski

1. Introduction

Urinary tract (UT), in its entirety, has a long and interesting history extending far beyond modern times. The first written mention of UT and especially kidneys reaches ancient Egypt, as kidneys together with the heart, were the only organs not removed from the mummified bodies [1]. It was believed that the kidneys are the means of judgment in the afterlife, the proverbial guide for the heart's decisions. The fundamental role of kidneys and heart for humans' afterlife fate was not only Egyptian domain as it was also a common belief among other ancient civilizations and religions, such as Semitic Tradition and Old Testament [2, 3].

The fact that the kidneys were not removed from dead bodies before mummification and burial has been the reason for today's existence of the archaic samples of those organs with, e.g., renal cysts and stones [1, 4]. As such, the knowledge of urinary tract infections (UTIs) also reaches ancient times. They were not called UTIs but were well defined nonetheless, together with very specific ways of treatment (e.g. [1]). The first written mention of UTI dates back again to ancient Egypt and the Ebers Papyrus from 1550 BC, where UTI is described as 'sending forth heat from bladder' [5]. It is worth underlining that the actual role of UT was far from correct in those ancient times, but still, the aforementioned Ebers Papyrus contains interesting descriptions of maladies such as urethritis, prostatitis, or cystitis and procedures such as uroscopy, which will be the modern urinalysis [1]. Later on, but still, in Antiquity, despite very limited and often quite erroneous knowledge of urinary tract functioning, Hippocrates and his successors were able to perform a rudimental urinalysis, noting such features as color, consistency, sediment, odor, and volume [6]. Corpus Hippocraticum presented many known renal afflictions today, such as renal colic, chronic renal infection, renal tuberculosis, and UTI symptoms, e.g., urinary incontinence and urinary retention [4].

The historical breakthrough for the UT elements and their role in physiology dates back to the brilliant scientist Galen of Pergamon, who was the first to claim and prove that the main role of kidneys, not the bladder, is to produce urine [7]. Even though the exact mechanism of urine formation remained a mystery to this scientist because the function was described as 'the separation of excess and poorly concocted bodily humors', the impact of Galen on nephrology cannot be diminished both in the case of uroscopy and the structure of the kidneys [7]. What is even more important, when it comes to Galen's impact on nephrology, is his contribution to its pathology. Galen is, e.g., credited for the first differential diagnosis and work-up of anuria and oliguria. His work also details the approach to a patient with such conditions as diabetes mellitus and diabetes insipidus, even though the exact pathomechanisms of those diseases themselves were a mystery at that time [8].

An even more detailed description of kidneys and UT was created by Oribasius from Pergamum, the Byzantine scholar who, apart from his impact on nephrology development, was remembered as the writer of *Collectiones Medicae* [4, 9], preserving the ancient medical knowledge. His descriptions of the nephron structure, together with a detailed illustration of its blood circulation, were the most detailed at the time. His proposed treatment options for hematuria, both acute and chronic nephritis and nephrolithiasis, even though they are not on par with today's practice, emphasized the role of physiotherapy and phytotherapy in nephropathology of that time [9]. Another Byzantine scholar – Avicenna – preserved the at the time known practices and knowledge from Greek and Far Eastern regarding urinalysis [10]. He said that 'urine is a faithful guide for the knowledge of the illness', which is a succinct description of the idea standing behind urinalysis.

2. Postantiquity advances in nephrology

Beginning from the Renaissance, the modern history of nephrology started. It still greatly drew from the knowledge of ancient scientists and physicians, in part mentioned above, but the new equipment allowed the previously unattainable precision in human anatomy and physiology observation [4]. Andreas Vesalius, the Belgian anatomist, and Roman Bartolomeo Eustachio working separately at more or less the same time, based their discoveries on direct observations of humans' and dogs' kidneys. Their meticulous work allowed them to correct many of the mistakes of their predecessors (and still, they had different results regarding some of the anatomical features of analyzed kidneys, e.g., the position of the right and left one in the human body) when it comes to the anatomy of the kidney [11]. Where Vesalius and Eustachio were quite ignorant of the function of the kidney itself [12], Neapolitan physicist and mathematician Giovanni Borelli was vitally interested in mechanisms explaining the mechanics of the body, among them kidney functioning, stating that the kidneys play the role of sieve filtering blood and excreting the elements which need to be eliminated [11]. Marcello Malpighi and Lorenzo Bellini, other renowned physicians, who were additionally armed with magnifying lenses and microscopes, were able to perform even more detailed observations of renal structure and function, especially Malpighians' body of the kidney [13]. Bellini, Borello, and Malpighi though, even with all the advances in their observations, still believed that urine is created in purely mechanistic or hydraulic ways [11, 14]. The concept of ultrafiltration as the means of urine formation was first described by Archibald Pitcairne, even though it was properly termed almost 150 years later [11]. The final touches to the kidney anatomy and function were added by William Bowman, who, armed with a microscope far better than Malpighi's and Bellini's described the existence of Bowman capsule surrounding the Malpighi's body. That in itself added the missing element to the urine formation hypothesis [15].

Richard Bright is considered the father of modern clinical nephrology. Together with other famous physicians, Thomas Hodgkin and Thomas Addison, they developed knowledge about specific pathologies; some were even named after them [4]. Bright discovered that the presence of albuminuria and edema is always linked with kidney disease [16]. He described such conditions as acute nephritis, nephrotic syndrome, and uremia. Additionally, he found and explained the link between kidney disease and enlarged ventricles of the heart [17].

Urinalysis remained largely unchanged at the time. As a visual science, it linked the observed changes in color, consistency, sediment, odor, and taste with specific diseases. And diabetes mellitus and diabetes insipidus are the best in proving the need for tasting the sample as the first means 'sweet as honey' and the second 'without taste or perceptible flavor' [18]. What is worth mentioning, though, is that with uroscopy becoming more and more popular, there were regions around the world where uromancy developed [19]. Many of those not knowledgeable enough made it a practice to diagnose various diseases based on information from pamphlets containing elaborate charts allowing comparing the color of the urine to diagnose assorted diseases [20]. Later on, it led to the need for uroscopy regulation, and some statutes were formulated trying to regulate the art of uroscopy [21].

3. The dawn of modern urinalysis

Together with the anatomical and functional advances of nephrology, also nephropathology and diagnostics started to develop. The autopsies of dead bodies brought many pathologies to light. Interesting results were revealed by, e.g., Malpighi's body autopsy [22]. He suffered from chronic kidney disease and supposedly hypertension, and his autopsy results were published together with over 2000 others in Theophile Bonet's *Sepulchretum sive anatomia practica ex cadaveribus morbo denatis*. The first such extensive collection of postmortem reports [22]. In turn *De Sedibus et Causis Morborum per anatomen indigatis* published almost 100 years later by Giovanni Morgagni, is considered the foundation for the classification of kidney diseases based on gross anatomy and clinical symptoms [23].

The development of physiology and pathology was accompanied by the advances in chemistry of urine. The first ones mentioning the exact parameters of urine, such as specific gravity, hematuria, or proteinuria, were Paracelsus and his two followers, Joan Baptista van Helmont and Herman Boerhaave [24, 25]. The chemistry knowledge in those days was not on par with physiology development though [26]. The dominant role of alchemy at the time had some impact on that. The beginning of actual urinalysis based on actual chemical structure is set in the seventeenth century. It was then that chemistry was freed from the influences of mystic alchemy and started to make headways. Many manuals were published about the principles of basic chemical methods, such as distillation and sublimation but also many others. Christofle Glaser, Nicolas Lemery, and aforementioned Herman Boerhaave should probably be mentioned as the ones (but not the only ones) who impacted chemistry the most at the time [25, 27]. The chemicals in the urine were divided into nonvolatile acidic residues, identified as chloride salts later on, and 'volatile alkali', ammonium carbonate, or urea. The aforementioned Bellini and Thomas Willis should probably be credited to be the ones of first authors of quite extensive descriptions of changes in urine (its' color, taste, and odor) depending on the urine's composition and clinical condition [18]. Willis was also the one involved in regulating uroscopy, mentioned earlier, by clearly stating that the observed changes in urine's color, taste, and odor reflect those of the blood, not mystic humors [28]. The link between blood and urine and the need to analyze them both to get a clear picture of various illnesses was also later underlined by others, e.g., Robert Boyle and Browne Langrish [25, 29]. The last one even said 'the study of the proportions of several principles of blood and urine, both in sound and disease state, will be highly useful in investigating the causes and the phenomenon of disease' [29].

The inauguration of biochemistry is dated to the beginning of the nineteenth century. Probably the most important milestone from that time is the identification of a vital element of urine – urea. It was identified and characterized by William Prout and synthesized by Friedrich Wöhler [30, 31]. Quite quickly, urea was linked with several pathologies, and the term 'uremia' was coined. The first disease in which an elevated level of serum urea was noted was mentioned earlier Bright's disease (or nephritis), but soon the urea level started to get measured in many other kidney diseases [32]. But what is most important about the research regarding urea is its role in the development of the concept of dialysis and artificial kidney [33].

The first complete compendium about the analysis of urine, *Quantitative Clinical Chemistry*, was published at the beginning of the twentieth century by John P. Peters and Donald D. Van Slyke [34]. It contained a detailed description of blood and urine chemical composition and the rules for standardized measurement of such parameters as electrolytes concentration, especially K^+, and Na^+. That allowed for assessing conditions such as hyponatremia, respiratory and metabolic acidosis, and effective osmotic pressure [35, 36]. As all of them are linked with renal state, Peters insisted on combining clinical laboratory and clinical investigation. That way, laboratory diagnostics became vital to clinical diagnosis [34]. By the end of the 30s of the 20th century, urinalysis started to become a common routine in medical examinations [37].

Almost 100 years later, urinalysis is still considered one of the most important tools implemented in standard medical examination. This period was filled with an intense development of that branch of the diagnostic laboratory. Many new techniques were developed, increasing the sensitivity and specificity of performed tests and making it easier to interpret obtained results even in specific and demanding groups of patients, e.g., pregnant women.

Author details

Agnieszka Daca[1*] and Tomasz Jarzembowski[2]

1 Department of Pathology and Experimental Rheumatology, Medical University of Gdansk, Gdansk, Poland

2 Deparment of Microbiology, Medical University of Gdansk, Gdansk, Poland

*Address all correspondence to: agnieszka.daca@gumed.edu.pl

References

[1] Salem ME, Eknoyan G. The kidney in ancient Egyptian medicine: Where does it stand? American Journal of Nephrology. 1999;**19**(2):140-147

[2] Diamandopoulos A, Goudas P. The role of the kidney as a religious, cultural and sexual symbol. American Journal of Nephrology. 2002;**22**(2-3):107-111

[3] Maio G. The metaphorical and mythical use of the kidney in antiquity. American Journal of Nephrology. 1999;**19**(2):101-106

[4] Greydanus D, Kadochi M. Reflections on the medical history of the kidney: From Alcmaeon of Croton to Richard bright – standing on the shoulders of giants. Journal of Integrative Nephrology and Andrology. 2016;**3**(4):101

[5] Easmon CFS. Topley & Wilson's principles of bacteriology, virology and immunity. Immunology. 1984;**52**(4):780

[6] Hippocrates AF. The Genuine Works of Hippocrates; translated from the Greek with a preliminary discourse and annotations [Internet]. New York: W. Wood; 2023. p. 416. Available from: http://archive.org/details/genuineworksofhi00tran

[7] Eknoyan G. The origins of nephrology – Galen, the founding father of experimental renal physiology. American Journal of Nephrology. 1989;**9**(1):66-82

[8] Temkin O. A Galenic model for quantitative physiological reasoning? Bulletin of the History of Medicine. 1961;**35**(5):470-475

[9] Eftychiadis AChr. Renal and glomerular circulation according to Oribasius (4th century). American Journal of Nephrology. 2002;**22**(2-3):136-138

[10] Abdel-Halim RES. The role of Ibn Sina (Avicenna)'s medical poem in the transmission of medical knowledge to medieval Europe. Urology Annals. 2014;**6**(1):1-12

[11] Eknoyan G. The scientific revolution—The kidney and nephrology in and about the seventeenth century (part 1). Seminars in Dialysis. 2015;**28**(3):282-292

[12] DeBroe ME, Sacreacute D, Snelders ED, De Weerdt DL. The Flemish anatomist Andreas Vesalius (1514-1564) and the kidney. American Journal of Nephrology. 1997;**17**(3-4):252-260

[13] McVaugh MR. Losing ground. The disappearance of attraction from the kidneys. The changing concepts of physiology from antiquity into Early Modern Europe. In: Blood, Sweat and Tears. The Netherlands: Brill; 2012. (Intersections; vol. 25)

[14] Brown TM. Medicine in the shadow of the principia. Journal of the History of Ideas. 1987;**48**(4):629-648

[15] Eknoyan G. Sir William Bowman: His contributions to physiology and nephrology. Kidney International. 1996;**50**(6):2120-2128

[16] Dock W. Proteinuria: The story of 280 years of trials, errors, and rectifications. Bulletin of the New York Academy of Medicine. 1974;**50**(6):659-666

[17] Young RH. Dr Richard bright – Father of medical renal disease. Archives of Pathology & Laboratory Medicine. 2009;**133**(9):1365

[18] Eknoyan G. Looking at the urine: The renaissance of an unbroken

tradition. American Journal of Kidney Diseases. 2007;**49**(6):865-872

[19] Armstrong JA. Urinalysis in Western culture: A brief history. Kidney International. 2007;**71**(5):384-387

[20] Wellcome HS et al. The Evolution of Urine Analysis: An Historical Sketch of the Clinical Examination of Urine: Lecture Memoranda. Los Angeles: American Medical Association; 1911. Available from: https://onlinebooks.library.upenn.edu/webbin/book/lookupid?key=ha002083175

[21] Pelling M, White F, Pelling M, White F. Medical Conflicts in Early Modern London: Patronage, Physicians, and Irregular Practitioners 1550-1640. Oxford, New York: Oxford University Press; 2003. p. 428. Oxford Studies in Social History

[22] Hajdu SI. The first printed treatise in pathology. Annals of Clinical and Laboratory Science. 2009;**39**(1):92-93

[23] Antonello A, Calò L, Bonfante L, Mennella G, Abaterusso C, Spinello M, et al. Giovan Battista Morgagni, a Pioneer of clinical nephrology. American Journal of Nephrology. 1999;**19**(2):222-225

[24] Bernoulli R. Paracelsus – physician, reformer, philosopher, scientist|SpringerLink. Experientia. 1999;**50**(4):334-338

[25] Fruton JS. The emergence of biochemistry. Science. 1976;**192**(4237):327-334

[26] Moran BT. Distilling Knowledge. USA: Harvard University Press; 2005. Available from: https://www.jstor.org/stable/j.ctvjz83pp

[27] Neville RG. Christophle Glaser and the 'Traité de la Chymie,' 1663. Chymia. 1965;**10**:25-52

[28] Eknoyan G, Nagy J. A history of diabetes mellitus or how a disease of the kidneys evolved into a kidney disease. Advances in Chronic Kidney Disease. 2005;**12**(2):223-229

[29] Foster WD. The early history of clinical pathology in Great Britain. Medical History. 1959;**3**(3):173-187

[30] Kinne-Saffran E, Kinne RKH. Vitalism and synthesis of urea: From Friedrich Wöhler to Hans a Krebs. American Journal of Nephrology. 1999;**19**(2):290-294

[31] Rosenfeld L. William Prout: Early 19th century physician-chemist. Clinical Chemistry. 2003;**49**(4):699-705

[32] Cameron J. Sir Robert Christison (1797-1882): The man, his times, and his contributions to nephrology. The Journal of the Royal College of Physicians of Edinburgh. 2007

[33] Gottschalk CW, Fellner SK. History of the science of dialysis. American Journal of Nephrology. 2008;**17**(3-4):289-298

[34] Seldin DW. Scientific achievements of John P. Peters. American Journal of Nephrology. 2002;**22**(2-3):192-196

[35] Bruckman FS, Peters JP. The plasma proteins in relation to blood hydration. The Journal of Clinical Investigation. 1930;**8**(4):591-595

[36] Peters JP, Wakeman AM, Eisenman AJ, Lee C. Total acid-base equilibrium of plasma IN health and disease. The Journal of Clinical Investigation. 1929;**6**(4):517-549

[37] Free AH, Free HM. Urinalysis, critical discipline of clinical science. CRC Critical Reviews in Clinical Laboratory Sciences. 1972;**3**(4):481-531

Chapter 2

Hospital-Acquired Urinary Tract Infections

Chandrasekhar Nagaraj

Abstract

Hospital-Acquired Infection (HAI/nosocomial infections) nosocomial infections, is gaining importance due to prolonged hospital stays and increased cost of hospital care as a result of infections acquired within the hospital. Organisms are more virulent and drug-resistant responsible for increased morbidity and mortality. Professor (Dr) Ignaz Phillip Semmelweis a Hungarian obstetrician, in 1847 observed this phenomenon. Catheter-associated Urinary Tract Infection (CAUTI) is the second most common infection (most common is Central Line-Associated bloodstream Infection–CLABSI). Development of CAUTI as an outcome, are discussed as pre-catheterization, input and output variable factors, and catheter maintenance. Careful monitoring is needed to understand these processes. **Pre-catheterization process** starts from the selection of the patient until catheterization is done. **Input variables** are catheter material, different types of urinary catheters, organisms causing these infections, and mechanism of infection. **Catheterization processes variables** include the need for catheterization, methods of catheterization, patient preparation, aseptic precautions, steps of catheterization, duration of catheterization, use of antibiotics, and the process of catheter removal. Final analysis of the cost involved makes it a comprehensive approach to the topic. Prevention of CAUTI as part of surveillance serves as an indicator to monitor the quality of services provided by the health care facility.

Keywords: hospital-acquired infection (HAI), nosocomial infections, urinary tract infection (UTI), catheter-associated urinary tract infection (CAUTI), asymptomatic bacteriuria, care bundle, health education, long-term catheter care, economic burden of hospitalization

1. Introduction

Catheter is a device used to drain urine from the bladder under different conditions. In the hospital, urinary catheters are used extensively on a variety of patient populations. During the process, the patient may get an infection other than for which he was admitted. In the hospital setup, urinary tract infection could follow the insertion of the urinary catheter. These infections following urinary catheterization are referred to as Catheter-associated urinary tract infection (CAUTI). CAUTI is a device (catheter) associated infection.

1.1 Urinary tract infections (UTIs)

Urinary tract infections (UTIs) are bacterial infections affecting nearly 150 million people around the world annually [1]. It is estimated that among all ambulatory patients (0.9%), 10.5 million persons have UTI symptoms and 2–3 million persons report to the emergency department in the United States alone [2–4]. In Infant boys, older men, and females of all ages, significant morbidity is due to UTIs. Frequent recurrences of pyelonephritis with sepsis, renal damage in young, preterm babies, and complications due to frequent antimicrobial use with high-level antibiotic resistance and Clostridium difficile colitis are the common complications of UTI. In the United States, approximately US$3.5 billion per year is spent on societal costs for UTI infections (includes health care costs and time missed from work).

Urinary catheterization is used to evacuate urine by passing a hollow catheter. Catheter is passed through the urethra or sometimes through the suprapubic region. Indwelling urinary catheterization is classified as short-term (*in situ* less than 28 days), or long-term (*in situ* greater than 28 days) based on the time interval the catheter is in place.

Clinically, UTIs are classified as uncomplicated or complicated. Uncomplicated UTIs affect individuals who are otherwise healthy with no structural or neurological urinary tract abnormalities [5, 6]. Uncomplicated UTI infections are again classified as cystitis (lower UTIs) and pyelonephritis (upper UTIs) [5, 7]. Risk factors associated with cystitis include female gender, a prior UTI, sexual activity, vaginal infection, diabetes, obesity, and genetic susceptibility [3, 7]. Complicated UTIs are associated with factors that compromise the urinary tract or host defense mechanisms, such as urinary obstruction, urinary retention (associated with neurological disease, immunosuppression, renal failure, renal transplantation, pregnancy and the presence of foreign bodies, including calculi, indwelling catheters or other drainage devices) [8, 9]. Indwelling catheters can be attributed to 70–80% of complications of UTIs [10], which translates to 1 million cases per year in the United States [4].

UTIs are caused by gram-negative bacteria, gram-positive bacteria, and by some fungi [11]. Uropathogenic *Escherichia coli* (UPEC) is the most common agent causing both uncomplicated and complicated UTIs. Other agents involved, in order of prevalence, causing uncomplicated UTIs are *Klebsiella pneumoniae*, *Staphylococcus saprophyticus*, *Enterococcus faecalis*, group B *Streptococcus* (GBS), *Proteus mirabilis*, *Pseudomonas aeruginosa*, *Staphylococcus aureus,* and *Candida spp* [3, 6, 11–13]. Similarly, complicated UTIs are caused by Enterococcus spp., *K. pneumoniae*, *Candida spp.*, *S. aureus*, *P. mirabilis*, *Ps. aeruginosa,* and GBS in order of prevalence following UPEC [9, 11, 14–16].

1.2 Health care-associated infections (HCAI)

By definition, "an infection that was not incubating at the time of admission is considered nosocomial if it develops in a patient who has been hospitalized for 48 to 72 hours or more." Health care-associated infections (HCAIs) are acquired by patients during their hospital stay [17]. Initially, the term HCAIs was referred only to the infections acquired by patients admitted to an acute-care hospital. At present, HCAI includes infections contracted in various healthcare settings, such as long-term care, family medicine clinics, home care, and ambulatory care, where patients get treated. HCAIs are infections that first appear 48 hours or more or within 30 days following hospitalization (can go up to 90 days for orthopedic implants) [18]. Adverse drug events (ADE), HCAIs and surgical complications are the most common types of complications seen in hospitalized patients [19–23].

Estimates of the Center for Disease Control and Prevention (CDC) nosocomial infections contribute 0.7 to 10.1% of deaths and cause 0.1 to 4.4% of all deaths occurring in hospitals. US Center for Disease Control and Prevention project a figure of 1.7 million hospitalized patients to acquire HCAIs annually and more than 98,000 of them die [24]. HCAIs are the common complications associated with hospital care and one of the top ten leading causes of death in the USA [25]. Seven out of the 100 hospitalized patients in advanced countries and ten in emerging countries acquire an HCAI [26]. In high-income countries, of the 5–15% hospitalized HCAI patients, 9–37% are admitted to intensive care units (ICUs) [27, 28]. Around 0.5 million episodes of HCAIs are diagnosed every year in ICUs alone [23, 29, 30]. ICU patients are critically ill, immuno-compromised, and susceptible to HCAIs [31, 32]. Nosocomial infections affect more than 1.6 million patients annually costing about $ 4.5 billion in the United States.

Hungarian obstetrician Professor (Dr) Ignaz Phillip Semmelweis, visualized that healthcare providers could transmit disease among themselves or to the patients. He was working in a Maternity Hospital in Vienna when he identified the mode of transmission and spread of puerperal sepsis. In 1847, he observed higher rates of maternal deaths among patients treated by obstetricians and medical students compared to those cared for by midwives. At that time, he found a pathologist while carrying out an autopsy on a patient with puerperal sepsis accidentally wounded with the scalpel and died of sepsis. Semmelweis wrote that “both scalpel and physician’s contaminated hands could transmit organisms to mothers during labor.” He introduced hand washing with chlorinated lime to be used by every staff working in that obstetric hospital. This practice brought a large improvement in maternal mortality rates [33]. Koch’s postulates published in 1890, “the germ theory of disease” gave validity to Semmelweis’ theory of transmission of disease from doctor to patient. Thus, Semmelweis became the first to describe HCAI and also provide intervention through hand hygiene [34].

The 2021 National and State HAI Progress Report [35] provided a detailed classification of different HAIs – “Central Line-Associated Blood Stream Infections (CLABSI), Catheter-Associated Urinary Tract Infections (CAUTI), Ventilator-Associated Events (VAE), Surgical Site Infections (SSI), Methicillin-Resistant *S. aureus* (MRSA) bloodstream events, and *Clostridioides difficile* (*C. difficile*) events.” The report provided details in the form of technical tables with additional statistics about HAIs.

The report included infection-specific standardized infection ratios (SIRs) to measure progress in reducing HAIs compared to the 2015 baseline time period [36]. SIR is the ratio of the observed number of infections (events) to the number of predicted infections for a summarized time period. The report also included the standardized utilization ratios (SURs), which measure the use of a device by comparing the number of observed device days to the number of predicted device days [37]. The risk adjustment methodology of 2015 national baseline is used to calculate the SIR and SUR metrics.

1.2.1 Catheter-associated urinary tract infection (CAUTI)

CAUTI risk factors include catheterization for long periods, female gender, older age, and diabetes [38]. High recurrence rates of antimicrobial resistance among uropathogens that resulted in increased economic burden to the patients were noted in patients suffering from CAUTI. Increased morbidity and mortality of catheter-associated UTIs (CAUTIs) are the common cause of secondary bloodstream infections.

Hospital-acquired infections (HAIs) are associated with the use of devices such as catheters, ventilators, central lines, etc. Major causes of HAIs is due to prolonged hospitalization, use of invasive devices, such as catheters and irrational use of antibiotics [39]. More than 30% of annual infections are seen in the critical care area of the hospital [24]. Among the device-associated hospital-acquired infections, Central line-associated bloodstream infections (CLABSIs) are the most common [40]. It is followed by catheter-associated urinary tract infections (CAUTIs) and ventilator-associated pneumonia (VAP) [41].

Indwelling urethral catheters account for about 80% of UTI [40]. Catheters may facilitate colonization of the urinary bladder due to poor catheter placement, prolonged catheterization, poor aseptic technique, poor hand hygiene, and poor asepsis of the urethral orifice opening. Hence, catheters are a common source of urinary tract infections [42]. Catheter placement is not directly associated with the development of UTIs.

Each patient, depending on age, comorbidities, and socioeconomic status the test result and frequency of a UTI can differ significantly. Gram-negative bacteria, such as *E. coli*, *Klebsiella spp.*, *P. mirabilis*, *Ps. aeruginosa*, and *Citrobacter spp.*, are the predominant isolates in urinary tract infections. Gram-positive bacteria, such as *S. aureus* and *Enterococcus species,* are the most common [43, 44].

A secondary hospital-acquired bloodstream infection may occur as post-catheter-associated urinary tract infection, (17% of nosocomial bacteremia from urinary tract infections) with an associated mortality of 10% [45]. Asymptomatic bacteriuria is the presence of a significant bacterial count, that is, $>10^5$ CFU/mL (Colony Forming Units/mL). In a well-collected urine sample with aseptic precautions from a patient who has asymptomatic, bacteriuria is commonly seen in clinical practice [46]. It is associated with low sequelae and low morbidity. In the majority of cases, it is self-limiting. In pregnant women, asymptomatic bacteriuria needs to be treated.

The urinary tract is usually sterile except for the distal urethra. The infection mostly follows instrumentation of the urinary tract, particularly catheterization (66–88%). Each case of hospital-acquired urinary tract infection adds approximately $675 to the cost of hospitalization, which increases to $2800 when bacteremia develops [47]. Patient mortality may be high (~30%) [48]. The incidence of hospital-acquired urinary tract infection can be reduced by decreasing the use of inappropriate indwelling urinary catheters, using closed drainage and ensuring the removal of the catheter when it is not required [49].

Leaving a urinary catheter for a long time *in situ* contributes to the development of a catheter-associated urinary tract infection (CAUTI) [50]. Risk of development of CAUTI increases by 5% per day in relation to the length of catheter *in situ*. Twenty-five percent of hospitalized patients are catheterized at some stage of their admission. It is critical to follow proper practices and procedures to minimize the risk of infection [51, 52].

A history of long-term hospitalization attributable to device-related infections should alert the possibility of CAUTI. Common symptoms are dysuria, fever (>38°C), urgency, frequency, dysuria without any cause, flank pain, supra-pubic pain, urinary urgency, and hematuria. Positive urinary cultures are expected if the patient has not consumed antibiotics prior to the sample collection. The presence of bacteria in the urine without these symptoms is due to colonization [49]. An increase in treatment costs and risk of lethality for patients are observed.

Bacteriuria signifies either colonization (asymptomatic bacteriuria) or infection. Bacteriuria can be found both in catheterized and non-catheterized patients. Of the patients with catheter *in situ* for more than 30 days, ~10–30% will develop bacteriuria compared to 1% of non-catheterized patients [53, 54]. Colonization rather than infection is associated with bacteriuria accounting for more than 90% of patients who are on the urinary catheter [55]. Diagnosis of CAUTI is not evidence-based [56]. Established laboratory criteria to differentiate between CAUTI and asymptomatic bacteriuria are not available. Clinicians rely on a combination of clinical signs and symptoms in addition to laboratory-confirmed bacteriuria to reach the diagnosis of CAUTI [57]. Clinical signs and symptoms of CAUTI are fever, new-onset confusion, loin, or suprapubic pain [56, 58]. Fever is the most frequently encountered symptom. However, the absence of fever does not rule out infection [57].

1.2.2 Morbidity and mortality associated with CAUTI

An increased morbidity, mortality, and length of hospitalization are associated with CAUTI [59–64]. In hospital-acquired bloodstream infection, CAUTI is the primary source of infection (8.5%) [65]. Bacteremia surveillance revealed 3.8% of cases to have resulted from CAUTI [66].

1.3 Etiology

Noncomplicated cystitis (86%) and up to 90% of noncomplicated pyelonephritis are mainly associated with *E. coli infection* [67]. Though *E. coli* is the most common infection, complicated UTIs have a more varied etiology. Other gram-negative bacilli like *Klebsiella*, *Citrobacter*, and *Enterobacter spp*. cause 11%; and *Ps. aeruginosa*, 8%. Gram-positive bacteria also are encountered in catheter-associated urinary tract infections (CAUTI) with D-group *Streptococci* causing 19% of them, and *S. aureus*, 4% associated with complications. Polymicrobial UTI cases represent 30% of complicated CAUTI. Other microorganisms such as yeasts cause 18% of UTIs. The significant appearance of *Ps. aeruginosa* in those of nosocomial origin along with extended-spectrum beta-lactamase (ESBL) and quinolone-resistant Enterobacteriaceae are encountered in those having healthcare-associated acquisition and secondary bloodstream infections [68].

Scottish Intercollegiate Guidelines Network (SIGN) recommends careful recording of associated localizing (loin or supra pubic tenderness) or systemic features of CAUTI. We have to exclude the possibility of other sources of infection. An appropriate sample of urine is to be sent for culture and the antimicrobial susceptibility of the organisms identified. An empiric antimicrobial therapy has to be considered based on the severity of the presentation, comorbid factors, and the local antimicrobial susceptibility patterns and antimicrobial prescribing guidelines [56].

1.4 Pathogenesis

Urethral catheterization interferes with the local natural defense mechanisms of the urinary tract. The length of the urethra and urine flow washes microorganisms away from the bladder. Most organisms that cause CAUTI have to enter the bladder by migrating along the internal (intraluminal) and external (extraluminal) catheter surfaces. Intraluminal migration occurs when there is contamination of the catheter lumen that can occur due to the failure of a closed drainage system or from contaminated urine in the drainage bag. Extra luminal migration of microorganisms occurs from the perineum that can occur at the time after insertion of the catheter or later by capillary action *via* the outer surface of the catheter [58]. Patient's flora in the perineum region or the hands of HCWs provides the common pathogens associated with CAUTI, which include *E. coli*, *Enterococcus spp*., *Pseudomonas spp*., *Klebsiella spp*., *Enterobacter spp*., or *Candida spp* [69]. Risk factors of CAUTI are the duration of catheterization [59, 70, 71], underlying predisposing neurological disease, [61] female gender, [71, 72] and diabetes mellitus [71]. The importance of virulence surface proteins such as Type 1 and Type 2 fimbriae and surface attachment proteins such as FimH has been shown to be important in UPEC organisms which have come to light in recent days [72]. Similarly, pathogenicity islands (PAIs) designated ICEPm1, papAH, papEF, fimH, fyuA, and traT genes contribute to genomic variability and virulence that have also been identified and studied [73].

2. Factors to be considered prior to the insertion of a urinary catheter

Catheterization is done to drain the urine from the bladder. The main cause of hospital-acquired urinary tract infection revolves around the process of insertion to removal of the catheter. Draining of the urine can be done not only by transurethral catheterization but also by other routes, such as suprapubic or external drainage, by using a condom. With catheter being a central point of infection, it is important to prioritize the need of catheterization and if it is possible to avoid catheterization. The above facts suggest the need to understand conditions where catheterization is required, and when it can be avoided. There is a need to understand the methods of catheterization for use in different situations. These factors are discussed with the help of available literature on each variable factor.

2.1 Indications for catheterization and can catheterization be avoided?

Urinary catheterization is indicated [74–77] to relieve acute urinary retention due to bladder outlet obstruction, for assessing the healing of an open sacral or perineum wounds, to assist in achieving patient immobilization due to unstable thoracic, lumbar spine, or pelvic fractures, to monitor urinary output in critically ill patients or when a patient is unable or unwilling to collect urine during prolonged surgical procedures with general or spinal anesthesia, during regional analgesia for labor and delivery, for instillation of drugs or during urology investigations and for patient comfort during end of life care. In spite of delineating the conditions requiring catheterization, a urinary catheter is inappropriate in 21–54% of catheterized patients [78–80].

CDC guideline highlights the importance of limiting the use of urinary catheters to reduce the risk of UTI [81]. European Prospective Investigation into Cancer and Nutrition (EPIC) guidelines also advocate the selected usage of urinary catheterization and highlight avoidance when possible [82].

The most important measure to prevent CAUTI is to limit the use of urinary catheters and leave them in place only for the period indications persist [75, 82]. Based on comprehensive risk assessment, evaluation and the expected duration of catheterization a decision is to be made regarding whether to catheterize and what type of catheter should be used. Consideration should be given to alternative management methods (e.g., condom) [83].

Urinary catheters are to be used only when indicated and should be removed at the earliest possible time. Complications associated with catheterization are infection, bacteremia, urethritis, urethral strictures, hematuria, and bladder perforation [84–87]. In practice, it is noted that indwelling urethral catheters are used when it is not indicated or remain *in situ* for a longer period than necessary [78, 79, 88].

As an alternative, the use of an external catheter (e.g., condom system) should be considered if clinically appropriate and practical.

Urinary catheters should not be used for the convenience of patient care. It should not be used for obtaining urine samples to perform diagnostic tests. Alternative methods include the use of external catheter (e.g., condom system) or intermittent catheterization.

2.2 Methods of catheterization

Catheterization could be external (condom system), or indwelling catheter (a) inserted either in a health care facility or (b) by the patients themselves (self-catheterization). Indwelling catheters are also further classified as (i) short-term (a duration of catheterization intended to be less than or equal to 14 days) or (ii) long-term (when a person uses a urinary catheter for at least four weeks, that is, for 28 days or more or (iii) intermittent indwelling catheters. The selection of method of catheterization should be decided on a patient basis.

Intermittent catheterization is advocated as a method of choice for patients with idiopathic or neurogenic bladder dysfunction due to residual urine in the bladder. Patients often experience urinary frequency, urgency, incontinence, and repeated urine infections [89]. Intermittent catheterization lower the rates of CAUTI as compared to urethral and suprapubic catheterization [75]. Greater patient independence, reduced interference with sexual activity and reduced need for equipment and appliances are the advantages [90].

Suprapubic catheterization is indicated for post-pelvic or urological surgery with difficulty in voiding, urethral trauma, chronic prostatitis, and post-gynecological surgery. Suprapubic catheterization is associated with lower rates of bacteriuria, re-catheterization, and urethral stricture [75].

3. Understanding the contributory factors OF CAUTI

The number of factors associated with the process of catheterization. With the available literature, individual factors are considered in the causation of urinary tract infections. Discussion of the variable factors could be studied as the material or the type of catheter used as input variable factors or the process of insertion to final removal as a process variable factor.

3.1 Input variable factors

Knowledge of different materials has accumulated in the field of material science, which has contributed to the development of a variety of catheters. These could be the use of different metals or antibiotic-incorporated catheters, which could prevent bacterial growth or nonirritant materials, which could prevent damage of the urethral epithelium, thus preventing breach of the surface of the urethral epithelial layer and thereby help in the retention of the catheter for a longer duration of time. These factors finally help the clinician to have a choice of the catheter to be used in different situations. Similarly, the length and size of the catheter are important factors to be considered.

3.1.1 Type of catheter

EPIC guidelines advocated the use of silver-coated catheters to reduce infection rates. This was not addressed in the earlier CDC guideline. A Cochrane Review concluded that the use of silver alloy indwelling catheters reduced the risk of CAUTI [91]. They recommended economic evaluation to confirm the reduction of infection.

Meta-analysis showed silver alloy-coated catheters to be significantly more effective in preventing bacteriuria [91–103]. Antimicrobial-coated catheters preventing catheter-associated bacteriuria/funguria during short-term catheterization were reported consistently [104]. However, no study demonstrated any clinical benefit for the use of different types of catheters.

3.1.2 Selection of a urinary catheter

Urinary catheters are of various types, sizes, and are made up of different materials. Foley's catheter is the most common type used. The Foley's catheter may have two or three lumens each of them with a different function to perform; one for the inflation of the balloon, second one for urine drainage of urine, and third one for irrigation.

3.1.3 Catheter size

Catheter size is measured by the diameter of the outer circumference (range from 6Fr-24Fr - French (Fr) metric scale). The smallest gauge that meets the needs of the patient should be the one to be given the choice of selection. It minimizes urethral trauma, reflux bladder spasm, and the amount of residual urine collected in the bladder. All these are predisposing factors to CAUTI [105, 106]. Catheters are manufactured in different lengths. The manufacturer's instructions are applicable [107].

3.1.4 Catheter material

Catheter material should be selected based on the patient's assessment and the clinician's preference. Duration of catheterization, patient comfort, patient history of allergies to the components (such as latex allergy), ease of insertion and removal, and the ability of the catheter material to reduce the likelihood of complications should decide the type of catheter material selected [108].

Commonly polyvinyl chloride (PVC), hydrogel, latex, silicone catheters, or a combination of these materials are used. Either latex or silicone-based catheters are the standard ones. Latex catheters are strong, elastic, and flexible and are common catheter types used for short-term catheterization. Silicone catheters (synthetic catheters) replace latex catheters in patients with latex sensitivity. There is no significant difference between the latex and silicone catheters and their contribution when it comes to the incidence of bacteriuria [85, 88, 109, 110]. For long-term use of catheters, evidence is insufficient to draw conclusions [111]. CDC advises the use of silicone catheters to reduce the risk of encrustation in long-term catheterized patients [75]. For intermittent catheterization, single-use catheters are preferred and are designed to be cleaned and reused. Manufacturers' instructions are to be followed strictly.

Antiseptic or antimicrobial-coated catheters are available with a variety of antimicrobial agents, such as gentamicin, [110] silver hydrogel, [93, 112] minocycline, rifampicin, [113] chlorhexidine-silver, sulfadiazine, chlorhexidine-sulfadiazine-triclosan, nitrofurazone, [113] and nitrofuroxone incorporated into the catheters [114]. Antiseptic or antimicrobial-coated catheters significantly prevent or delay the onset of CAUTI [110]. The poor quality of the studies makes decision-making difficult. Silver alloy catheters appear to be associated with a reduced incidence of bacteriuria [74, 115–119]. A Cochrane Review suggests the use of silver-alloy catheters used for less than one week [93]. The review also showed that antibiotic-impregnated catheters had lower rates of asymptomatic bacteriuria at less than one week of catheterization. When catheterization exceeded one week, the results were not statistically significant. Studies are needed to evaluate cost–benefit effectiveness of antiseptic and antimicrobial-coated catheters [77, 110].

3.2 Process variables

3.2.1 Use of aseptic (standard) precautions during urinary catheterization

To minimize the risk, HCWs are to be trained to perform catheterization and have to be assessed. Their competency in technical aspects and application of the principles of aseptic technique should be documented [74, 110, 120, 121].

Standard precautions "***must be applied by all HCWs for all patients at all times.***" They are useful to contain transmissible microorganisms that may be present in blood and body fluids, excretions, and secretions (except sweat). Standard precautions "***must be applied by all HCWs for all patients at all times***" while performing close activities with patients, patients' surroundings, and handling and disposing clinical waste [122]. HCWs should wear sufficient personal protective equipment (PPE) to prevent skin or clothing contamination. Contaminated body fluids may contain pathogenic microorganisms which may get transferred either to themselves or other patients. While performing urinary catheter insertion, a disposable plastic apron, and sterile gloves will usually be sufficient [110, 122]. Disposable plastic aprons and gloves are single-use items that are to be worn and then discarded after each procedure [122]. Hands should be decontaminated before the procedure, after the procedure, and also after removing PPE [123].

3.2.2 Aseptic technique

During the insertion of indwelling and intermittent urinary catheters, HCWs must practice strict aseptic techniques and use sterile equipment as per the expert opinion, clinical guidance, and principles of best practice [124–128].

The aseptic technique refers to the practices that help to reduce the risk of post-procedure infections. This decreases the likelihood of microorganisms entering the body during clinical procedures. The aseptic technique reduces the risk of infection by preventing the transmission of microorganisms either directly or indirectly. Wide variations in the practice of aseptic techniques have been found in different surveys. A standardized aseptic non-touch technique (ANTT)™ has been developed [129].

3.2.3 Hand decontamination

Hand hygiene is the single most important procedure. The World Health Organization (WHO) advocates five situations (moments) of hand hygiene performance: [129] (a) Before touching the patient, (b) before a clean or aseptic procedure, (c) after body fluid exposure risk, which also includes emptying a urinary catheter drainage system [125, 130], (d) after touching the patient's surroundings, and (e) after touching the patient. Except when an aseptic procedure is being performed, non-sterile single-use gloves should be worn. Hands should be decontaminated before and after removing PPE [124, 125, 130].

3.2.4 Patient preparation

Patients should be provided with adequate information regarding the need for catheter insertion, catheter maintenance, and removal of the catheter by the caregiver. The patient should be given the opportunity to discuss the implications of the procedure [120].

3.2.4.1 Skin/meatus cleaning and disinfection

Patient preparation to prevent infection during catheterization depends on the method of catheterization, skin or meatus cleaning and disinfection. This process is also carried out for daily maintenance of the catheter.

3.2.4.1.1 Meatus cleaning prior to catheterization

As infection can get transmitted *via* the external surface of the catheter during catheter insertion especially when an indwelling or intermittent catheter is used. Here, the urethral meatus should be cleaned prior to catheterization [77], which involves the mechanical removal of exudate and smegma washing the meatus area with soap and water [128]. The use of antiseptic solution versus sterile saline wash prior to catheter insertion needs more evidence [64, 108, 131–134].

The standard practice of cleansing the urethral meatus is to retract the foreskin (where possible), cleaning the glans penis, and return the foreskin to normal position after insertion of the catheter. A front-to-back cleaning technique should be adopted after the labia minora are separated for women. After a thorough cleaning, the urethral opening should be washed and cleaned with sterile water or sterile saline solution. The area should be wiped dry using sterile swabs. The gauze ball or swab should be discarded after a single use. The same procedure is to be performed before self-intermittent catheterization.

3.2.4.1.2 Suprapubic catheterization

The skin over the insertion site should be washed with soap and water. Then, the site is dried thoroughly. Then, it is cleaned with an aqueous or alcohol-based surgical site disinfectant solution (e.g., chlorhexidine or povidone-iodine) as per local guidelines [135].

3.2.5 Maintaining a sterile field

Before each procedure, environmental surfaces should be effectively cleaned and disinfected as practiced for any other minor surgical procedure [136]. Maintaining the integrity of the sterile field is important. HCWs should use sterile gloves and a drape to create a sterile field [74]. Sterile catheter packs, which contain all needed materials should be used [110].

3.2.6 Steps of catheterization

Steps of catheterization start from the process of insertion till the catheter is removed. Since infection could occur at any step of catheterization, each of them are analyzed with the available scientific data.

3.2.6.1 Catheter insertion

The CDC guideline stresses that catheters should be inserted using sterile equipment and an aseptic technique [81]. The use of aseptic technique was not shown to reduce CAUTI in a systematic review, [137] and following principles of good practice, clinical guidance [81, 138], and expert opinion [119, 139–142]. However, the EPIC guidelines concluded that urinary catheters must be inserted aseptically [82].

In a study focused on the influence of sterile versus clean technique for catheter insertion found no statistical difference between the two groups, while there was a considerable cost difference [143]. The sterile method was found to be more than twice as expensive as the clean method. It was concluded that strict sterility was not necessary for preoperative short-term urethral catheterization.

3.2.6.2 Insertion procedure

3.2.6.2.1 Indwelling urethral catheterization

The entry point for microorganisms into the blood and lymphatic system was a bruise or trauma to the urethral mucosa that occurred during catheterization [144]. To minimize urethral trauma and infection, it is recommended to apply sterile lubricant or anesthetic gel from a single-use container [110]. Once the catheter is inserted, urine is allowed to drain and the balloon is inflated to secure the catheter in place. The indwelling catheter is then connected to a closed sterile drainage bag, which is placed below the level of the bladder to facilitate drainage.

Documentation of the patient information is recorded, which includes an indication for catheter insertion, date and time of catheter insertion, type and size of catheter, amount of water used to inflate the balloon, any complications encountered, review date and name of HCW who inserted catheter [145].

3.2.6.2.2 Intermittent catheterization

Intermittent catheterization is affected by the use of sterile or clean technique, coated or uncoated catheters, single (sterile) or multiple-use (clean) catheters, self-catheterization or catheterization by others, or by any other strategy that need further clarification [89]. Many guidelines recommend an aseptic technique and sterile equipment for intermittent catheterization in a healthcare setting. A clean technique is recommended for self-intermittent catheterization [75, 110, 145].

3.2.6.2.3 Suprapubic catheterization

Suprapubic catheter is commonly done in a theater by a urologist/surgeon, with all sterile precautions. Some catheters are secured to the abdominal wall by a suture. A small sterile dressing may be placed over the site, which can be removed after 24 hours.

3.2.6.3 Catheter maintenance and dwell time

The CDC guideline addresses adherence to a sterile closed system as the cornerstone of infection control. Irrigation should be avoided unless there is a need to prevent or relieve the obstruction [81]. The EPIC guidelines state that a sterile, continuously closed urinary drainage system is central to the prevention of CAUTI [121]. The use of a closed urinary drainage system is effective [126, 140, 141, 146–150].

The CDC guidelines [82] stress the need to avoid meatus care using povidone-iodine. The EPIC guidelines, based on expert opinion [81, 140, 141] and one systematic reviews [74] recommend against vigorous meatus cleansing. The EPIC guideline recommends daily routine bathing or showering to maintain meatus hygiene [82, 117]. In three earlier studies that investigated meatus care to prevent bacteriuria, little or no benefit was found other than standard personal hygiene in patients with indwelling catheters [151–153].

The literature review concluded that flushing catheters and daily perineum care do not prevent infection [147].

Only one study which examined different types of catheters showed that substances in the latex urinary catheter were toxic to *E. coli* [88].

There is a direct relationship between dwell time and incidence of infection [81, 149, 154–156]. Urinary tract catheterization of at least 3 days was sufficient to increase the risk of urinary tract infection [97]. Early removal is key to the prevention of UTI [77, 151, 157, 158]. Early removal is also associated with shorter hospital stays [91, 155].

3.2.6.4 Catheter removal

Neither the CDC nor the EPIC guidelines discuss catheter removal. Best strategies for the removal of catheters were reviewed through 26 trials involving a total of 2933 participants [155]. Inconclusive evidence of the benefit for midnight removal of indwelling catheters and the need for re-catheterization have been noted. There is only a little evidence for the effectiveness of catheter clamping [91].

4. Management of urinary catheters

Care of drainage system needs proper care for infection prevention. Care of urinary bag, catheter position, and handling of the wound are important in infection prevention.

4.1 Drainage systems

Urinary drainage is done through a catheter connected to a drainage tube, which opens into a drainage bag. In a closed system, the catheter is to be connected to the drainage tube and that is not disturbed. Urine is emptied into the bag through a valve or a port that reduces the risk of ascending infection from intraluminal transmission. Irrespective of the drainage system, daily care is needed to prevent infection. Its effectiveness is dependent on good catheter hygiene [77, 82, 109, 136, 159, 160]. Closed system is the best method to manage the drainage system to prevent CAUTI [110, 117].

4.1.1 Drainage bags

Four main types of drainage bags are used with indwelling catheterization. A leg drainage bag with a drainage tap directly attached to the catheter, a drainage bag with a drainage tap secured to a catheter stand, a non-drainable bag with no drainage tap which is secured to a catheter stand (useful for overnight drainage), and a combined drainage bag and urinary catheter, which is pre-connected to the catheter during the manufacturing process.

4.1.2 Management of catheterized patients

For catheterized patients with spinal cord injury and patients admitted to long-term care facilities advocate reusing drainage bags after cleaning and disinfection is advocated (Best practice guidelines) [160, 161]. It does not increase the risk of CAUTI [161–163]. This practice is an unacceptable procedure since it does not provide a validated method for decontamination [164, 165]. This practice is not discussed in other evidence-based guidelines [74, 76, 77, 110, 117]. The recommendation is for the use of single-use drainage bags.

Sterile and non-sterile (i.e., clean) drainage bags are available in the market. A sterile bag is used for directly connecting the bag to the catheter which is accepted by evidence-based guidelines [74, 75, 83, 110, 162]. Non-sterile Catheters are used in some healthcare settings [165]. No studies comparing the CAUTI rate with sterile and non-sterile night drainage bags were available in the literature and require further studies. The use of pre-connected urinary catheters and drainage bags reduces the risk of CAUTI [166]. However, there is no conclusive data [75, 77, 166–168].

A good practice is to maintain the bag below the level of the bladder, [136, 169] minimize contamination of the drainage bag outlet port by avoiding contact with the floor or other surfaces, [136, 159] access the catheter drainage system only when absolutely necessary (e.g., changing the drainage bag as per the manufacturer's instructions), [80] empty the drainage bag regularly to prevent reflux and use a separate clean container for each patient and prevent the container touching the drainage tap when emptying the drainage bag [80, 98].

4.2 Collecting catheter specimens of urine (CSU)

A sampling port is made available for the collection of urine samples. The sampling port should be disinfected with an appropriate disinfectant (e.g., 70% alcohol) and allowed to dry fully before collecting the sample. Manufacturer's instructions should be followed. Single-step, needle-free urine collection containers that are suitable for laboratory use should be used to reduce HCW exposure to urine splash and needle stick injuries [170].

4.3 Catheter valves

A catheter valve is a device connected to the end of the catheter and its value is being evaluated. The catheter valve allows urine to be stored in the bladder and eliminates the need for a urine drainage bag. The valve is released at regular intervals to prevent over-distension of the bladder or dilation of the renal tract. The catheter valves may reduce the risk of CAUTI, [171–173] reduce bladder irritation [172] and maintain bladder tone and capacity. This helps to improve the rehabilitation process after catheter removal.

Evidence suggests that patients prefer to use the catheter valves [157]. But the use of a catheter valve is contraindicated in patients with limited bladder capacity, [174] reflux or renal impairment, [173] detrusor muscle instability, [165, 166] mental disorientation, [171] impaired bladder sensation, [171] poor manual dexterity [175], and immobility.

4.4 Securing indwelling urethral catheters

Use of adhesive, nonadhesive devices (e.g., elastic/Velcro® straps) to secure the urinary catheter to the leg, or abdomen is recommended (best practice guidelines and expert opinion) [75, 169, 175, 176]. By securing the catheters, trauma and bleeding are reduced, dislodgement is prevented and bladder spasms, which may result from pressure and traction are also prevented. These are seen as advantages [177, 178]. A systematic literature review [178] has shown no evidence suggestive of catheter-securing system capable of preventing CAUTI. Though no statistically significant differences were found, the clinical significance of 45% reduction in the rate of symptomatic UTI was noted in patients who received the securing device [179].

It is recommended to place the securement device at the stiffest part of the catheter (usually just below the bifurcation where the balloon is inflated) to prevent occlusion of the lumen. The securement device can be placed on the abdomen or thigh [176]. To prevent skin trauma from excess traction, a regular assessment is necessary. In addition, adhesive material may result in skin irritation and dermatitis and elasticized / Velcro® straps should be used with caution, especially in patients with peripheral vascular disease [176, 180]. The skin site used for the securing device should be regularly changed.

4.5 Suprapubic catheters

The suprapubic catheter emerges at right angles to the abdomen. It needs to be secured in this position. Dressing and tapes should only be used on the healed insertion site when it is absolutely necessary.

4.6 Meatus and insertion site care

4.6.1 Indwelling urethral catheters

There is no advantage in using antiseptic preparations for meatus care over routine bathing or showering [136, 144, 181, 182]. Vigorous meatus cleansing beyond normal hygiene practice is not recommended. It may increase the risk of infection. Washing the meatus with soap and water during daily routine bathing or showering is all that is required. If this forms part of a bed bath, the water should be changed and a clean cloth should be used [183]. Prevention of contamination of the entry site of the catheter during cleaning is important. For women adopting a front-to-back approach, washing toward the anus is to be practiced. For uncircumcised men, the foreskin should be retracted before the area underneath is cleaned. This is often a reservoir for bacteria, particularly in the elderly [169].

4.6.2 Suprapubic catheter

An aseptic technique with a suitable cleansing solution and a sterile dressing should be used for wound care until the insertion site is healed [145]. Once healed, the site should be washed daily with warm water and soap.

4.7 Catheter irrigation

There is no evidence to suggest routine irrigation of a urinary catheter. Using antiseptic or antimicrobial agents to decrease CAUTI has no place in the management [10, 121]. A closed continuous irrigation system should be used if irrigation is required for other reasons (e.g., post-surgery). An aseptic technique should be used for intermittent irrigation (e.g., flushing or installation of drugs).

4.7.1 Catheter blockage

Each patient should have an individualized care regimen designed to minimize the problems of blockage and encrustation. The recurrent blockage is due to the encrustation of the catheter from mineral salt deposits. It is a complication in approximately 50% of all long-term catheterized patients [184]. Catheter blockage causes leakage, bypassing of urine and urinary retention. This condition results in the increased number of catheter changes. Encrustation on the external surface can cause trauma to the urethra during catheter removal.

Catheter maintenance solutions (CMS) are acidic washout solutions. CMS is commonly used to prolong catheter life by reducing pH, which helps in the dissolution of existing encrustations [82]. Disruption of the closed system increases the risk of infection. Frequent blockage leads to frequent re-catheterization. Potential infection risks associated with CMS use are outweighed by increased catheter life and reduced patient discomfort [185]. HCWs should be alert for the signs and symptoms of autonomic dysreflexia in patients with spinal cord injuries. Autonomic dysreflexia is a life-threatening condition.

4.8 Catheter removal

The risk of acquiring bacteriuria has been estimated at 5% for each day of catheterization, accumulating to 100% in 4 weeks. The longer the catheter remains *in situ*, higher is the risk of infection [133]. Catheterization should be reviewed daily and removed as soon as possible [75, 121, 182]. Clamping urinary catheters prior to removal is not to be followed [75].

4.8.1 Strategies for limiting the duration of short-term catheters

Success strategy in limiting catheter use and duration of catheterization is achieved by implementing procedure-specific guidelines for postoperative catheter removal, and providing reminders to physicians to review and limit the duration of catheterization [186–190]. Providing guidelines to manage postoperative retention may include the use of bladder scanners [187]. Care plans/protocols directing nurses to remove catheters need to be developed [187, 189, 191].

The effectiveness of reminder systems has helped in reducing CAUTI and urinary catheter use. Rate of re-catheterization was reduced by 52% following the use of reminder or stop orders. Duration of catheterization decreased by 37% and re-catheterization rates were similar in control and intervention groups, respectively [192].

4.8.2 Changing long-term catheters

Long-term catheterization is defined as a catheter *in situ* for greater than 28 days. No consensus exists on how frequently such catheters need to be changed. Manufacturer's instructions should be followed in addition to individual patient's requirements (e.g., before blockage occurs or is likely to occur) [76].

4.8.3 CAUTI preventive care bundles

Care bundles are useful in identifying the cause of CAUTI in each patient due to a breach in the process of catheter care. It analyses the clinical, laboratory, bacteriological, and radiological data and through root cause analysis (RCA) suggest corrective and preventive actions (CAPA) needed to prevent CAUTI infection. It follows the surveillance activity.

"A care bundle is a group of evidence-based practices that improve the quality of care." Care bundles have been developed for a range of conditions and disease processes [193–196]. Implementation of care bundles is helpful in improving the care of all patients in both multidisciplinary teams and individual wards/units. The decrease is significant when adjusted for device utilization [197].

Compliance with a care bundle for an individual patient is measured as either 100% or 0%. To achieve 100%, all of the evidence-based components of the bundle must be implemented. If one of the components of the care bundle is not in place, a score of zero is allocated. The ward or team score is calculated as the percentage of all patients with a urinary catheter that achieved 100% compliance with the care bundle.

4.9 Antimicrobial prophylaxis

There is no role for routine antimicrobial prophylaxis. Prophylaxis after the change or instrumentation of urinary catheters (both short and long-term) is not indicated. Despite a lack of evidence, the use of prophylactic antimicrobial (aminoglycosides are commonly used). This has resulted in overuse and increased resistance to antibiotics. The benefits of antimicrobial prophylaxis must be balanced against possible adverse effects like selection pressure for the development of antibiotic-resistant bacteria. C. difficile infection and antimicrobial toxicity are the other two effects of prophylactic overuse. Risk–benefit analysis cannot be reliably estimated. The effectiveness of prophylactic antimicrobials at the time of urinary catheter insertion, change, or removal is variable. There is a specific need for guidelines to be established [198].

All reviews showed limited evidence for the use of prophylactic antibiotics for both short-term and long-term catheters [155, 199]. Majority of best practice guidelines do not recommend the use of prophylactic antimicrobials before the removal of catheters. A comprehensive review also did not show any conclusion [200]. There is also little data regarding the patient with a previous episode of septicemia associated with catheter manipulations. The use of short-term catheterization to prevent bacteriuria appear to be a better strategy than the use of antimicrobials.

The asymptomatic bacteremia rate is approximately 10% per catheter change. It is unwise to recommend the use of prophylactic antimicrobials for long-term catheterized patients [200, 201]. Recently published guidelines from the US do not recommend the routine use of systemic antimicrobials at the time of catheter placement, removal, or replacement. According to CDC, unless clinical indications exist (e.g., in patients with bacteriuria upon catheter removal post-urologic surgery), routine use of systemic antimicrobials is not required.

UK National Institute for Health and Clinical Excellence (NICE) guidelines on antimicrobial prophylaxis against infective endocarditis also does not support the use of antibiotic prophylaxis to prevent endocarditis in patients undergoing urological procedures, including catheterization [202]. The British Society for Antimicrobial Chemotherapy state that the risk of bacteremia increases in presence of bacteriuria. Hence, treatment is recommended for pre-procedures [203]. US guidelines on the prevention of infective endocarditis, state that no published data is available to demonstrate a conclusive link between procedures of the gastrointestinal or genitourinary tract to be related to the development of endocarditis [204].

Prophylactic use of antimicrobials has no relation to change or instrumentation of urinary catheters (both short and long-term). In patients with bacteriuria, high risk of endocarditis or significantly immune compromised (e.g., patients with neutropenia, hematological malignancy, post solid organ transplantation), definitive randomized-controlled trials are needed.

5. Surveillance for CAUTI

Surveillance is "the ongoing systematic collection, analysis, and interpretation of data and the timely dissemination of the data to those who need to know to prevent and control infection" [205]. Prevalence studies are used to do surveillance of CAUTI [206–208]. Prospective CAUTI surveillance is useful for high-risk groups: (e.g., patients admitted to intensive care surgical or obstetric units) [10]. Rates of CAUTI range from 3.3 to 17.4/1000 catheter days among ICU patients [209–212]. Much lower infection rates (1.24–2.26/1000 catheter days) are reported in long-term care institutions [213]. Including CAUTI as part of the hospital's regular surveillance program should be considered by all hospitals depending on the risk profile of their patients and available resources. CAUTI rate should be reported as the number of CAUTI per 1000 urinary catheter days.

5.1 CAUTI definition for surveillance

The CDC or the HELICS definitions are most commonly used for HCAI surveillance [214, 215]. HELICS definition of urinary tract infection is specifically designed for use in intensive care units only. CDC definitions are to be used in acute facilities. CAUTI surveillance should only include symptomatic CAUTI, as the prevalence of asymptomatic bacteriuria is high among elderly care residents [216].

5.2 Forms and protocol for data collection

Data collectors should be trained in the definitions, surveillance, and protocols to be utilized. An example of data collection forms for CAUTI surveillance needs to be standardized and used.

Calculation of the denominator: Denominator value data is collected in this form. This is a daily count of all the urinary catheters in the area/patient group under surveillance. The number of patients with urinary catheter device *in situ* is known as urinary catheter days. Data should be collected at a specified time each day.

Calculation of the numerator: The numerator data is collected in this form. It represents the number of patients with CAUTI. This form is used to collect and report each suspected or confirmed CAUTI in the area/patient group under surveillance. Additional information that is to be collected includes patient demographics, signs and symptoms of infection, laboratory results if applicable and the presence or absence of a urinary catheter.

The CAUTI rate per 1000 catheter days is calculated by using the following formula:

$$\frac{\text{No of CAUTIs}}{\text{No. of U. Catheter days (denominator)}} \times 1000$$

Example: Calculation of CAUTI rate per 1000 catheter days.

1. One patient in the ICU met the case definition of a CAUTI in the month of January (numerator = 1).

2. To calculate the number of catheter days (denominator data); add the number of patients with a urinary catheter *in situ* on each day in the month of January (e.g., 4 patients on the first day of January had a urinary catheter *in situ*; 6 on day 2; 5 on days 3 to 8, 6 on days 9 to 16, 4 on day 17 to 23 and 7 on days 24 to 31 (4 + 6+ 5 + 5 + 5 + 5 + 5 + 5 + 6 + 6 + 6 + 6 + 6 + 6 + 6 + 6 + 4 + 4 + 4 + 4 + 4 + 4 + 4 + 7 + 7 + 7 + 7 + 7 + 7 + 7 + 7 = 144).

   144 = denominator data (number of catheter days in the month of January in the ICU).

3. The CAUTI rate for the month of January in the ICU (per 1000 urinary catheter days) is thus:

$$\frac{1 \times 1000}{144} = 6.9 \text{ CAUTIs/1000 catheter days}$$

CAUTI surveillance should be a part of routine hospital surveillance.

5.3 Surveillance result feedback

Regular CAUTI rate feedback to the relevant area(s) of the healthcare facility is very important along with any comments or suggestions for improvement. Ideally, it is monthly or at least once in a quarter. Feedback helps the healthcare facility to monitor the trends, identify outbreaks, and in addition to monitor the effectiveness of preventative programs.

6. Clinical presentation

Clinically, CAUTI presents with fever, new-onset confusion, loin, or suprapubic pain. Fever, though the most common symptom, absence of fever does not rule out infection. The Scottish Intercollegiate Guidelines Network (SIGN) recommends follow-up of catheterized patients with fever to be looked for associated localizing loin or suprapubic tenderness or systemic features, exclude other sources of infection, send an appropriate sample of urine for culture, consider empiric antimicrobial therapy as required by clinical presentation and severity and existing comorbid factors if any. Local antimicrobial susceptibility patterns and antimicrobial prescribing guidelines should be the guide for the suggestion of empirical treatment [56–58].

7. Laboratory findings

Bacteria in urine (bacteriuria) signifies either colonization (asymptomatic bacteriuria) or infection. Bacteriuria is detected in both catheterized and non-catheterized patients. An un-centrifuged sample of urine shows plenty of WBCs with motile or nonmotile bacteria on microscopic examination of urine. It is significant to note that in patients with catheter *in situ* greater than 30 days, 10–30% will develop bacteriuria compared to 1% of non-catheterized patients [53, 54]. More than 90% of catheter-associated bacteriuria are cases of colonization rather than infection [55]. Definitive diagnosis of CAUTI is not evidence based [56]. Laboratory criteria for differentiating between CAUTI and asymptomatic bacteriuria have not been established. The use of molecular techniques for not only diagnosis of CAUTI but also for antibiotic sensitivity for treatment may become important in the present scenario. Multiplexed RTPCR probes can be prepared and would be used in these situations. LAMP is another technology that is useful. Pathogenic bacteria can be tested for virulence using specific PCR probes and by surface active proteins known as adhesion proteins [72, 73].

A UTI can be tested by routine urine examination for the presence of bacteria, and inflammatory cells. This could be followed by culture and sensitivity for testing their sensitivity to different antimicrobials. With modern tools, phenotypic and genotypic expressions could be analyzed. Same time secondary bloodstream infections with the same organism detected in the urine could be noted. Their phenotypic and genotypic expression would give the possibility of selection for antibiotic sensitivity or secondary infection with a hospital-acquired organism could be identified. Molecular tools could be helpful in HAI surveillance of CAUTI.

8. Health education and training of HCWs

All HCWs and caregivers require education regarding the insertion and the removal of urinary catheter to prevent infection in the hospital setup. This is a continuous process and should be conducted at regular intervals. A similar education regarding the urinary catheter is to be given to the relatives and patient carers regarding the need for catheterization, catheter maintenance, chance of patient developing CAUTI, and importance of catheter care and how long the patient needs catheterization. They also need to be trained in meatus care with bathing, use of soap and water, and aseptic procedures used. This is not only an education to maintain the catheter in home care, intermittent and self-catheterization but also to induce confidence among the care givers.

8.1 Education for healthcare workers

A number of studies have demonstrated staff education programs can reduce HCAI [217, 218]. Best practice guidelines recommend staff education as a key factor in preventing CAUTI [10, 75, 110, 117, 181]. Education is a continuous process. It is to be done compulsorily at the time of induction of new staff. It should also become a regular education for HCWs. An induction education program should provide information regarding indications for catheterization, safe insertion technique, catheter maintenance, catheter removal, obtaining a urine specimen, and signs and symptoms of urinary infection. Attendance records of education sessions should be maintained.

The retraining education program should include technical topics, such as indications for catheterization, management of catheters, and removal of catheters, when no longer required. Some deficits in the knowledge and practice of HCWs have been identified.

The deficits in knowledge form the need for the next training. Some of the training needs identified include inappropriate use of a drainage tap to collect urine samples, [219] inappropriate use of lubricants for insertion, [220] daily changing of catheter bags [220], and poor documentation of the process [82, 221].

8.2 Education for patients/relatives/carers

Appropriate education of patients, relatives, and carers should focus on the management of urinary catheters, so that they can take part during home care [10, 75, 110, 119]. They should be trained for intermittent catheterization, insertion technique, and care of reusable catheters where appropriate. Support should be available for the entire duration of the catheterization [83].

Well-designed and appropriately written patient educational materials can augment other educational efforts, which ultimately improve patient care [222, 223]. These patient information leaflets should have a description of catheter care, emptying the catheter bag, when the catheter and catheter bag requires to be changed, signs and symptoms of complications (e.g., infection, leakage, and blockage), and whom to contact should complications develop.

9. CAUTI prevention

Numerous guidelines to prevent CAUTI highlight the importance of educational measures for all healthcare professionals [51]. Hand hygiene is the most important preventive step. If a patient is found to be colonized or infected, contact precautions along with a good environmental cleaning to avoid the Multi-Drug Resistant (MDR) organism transmission should be emphasized.

Unnecessary catheter insertion should not be encouraged. Reducing the period of catheterization is a relevant prevention strategy [78].

In a prospective study, initial indication was judged to be inappropriate in 21%, and continued catheterization was judged to be inappropriate for almost one-half of catheter days [80]. Surveillance is important [224]. A nationwide study showed 56% of hospitals were not having a system for monitoring and 74% did not monitor the duration of catheterization. A French prospective interventional study showed a reduction in CAUTI from 10.6 to 1.1 episodes per 100 patients when nurses and physicians were reminded daily to remove unnecessary urinary catheters four days after insertion [154]. It also decreased the incidence of CAUTI from 12.3 to 1.8 per 1000 catheter days. Alternative prevention strategies (use of antimicrobial-coated catheters, catheter irrigation with antimicrobials, antimicrobials in the drainage bag, or prophylaxis with cranberry products) can also be considered but they need more studies. In conclusion, simple practices, such as hand hygiene, limited and judicious use of catheters, and the use of some preventive additive procedures, can prevent CAUTI.

10. Treatment

Treatment of asymptomatic bacteriuria is needed only in pregnant women, before transurethral resection of the prostate or any traumatic genitourinary procedures associated with mucosal bleeding, in immunosuppressed patients, or after the first year of renal transplantation [225]. Treating nonpregnant women is to be considered if there is asymptomatic bacteriuria in the first 48 hours after urinary catheterization. In other cases, antibiotics only eliminate bacteriuria transitorily. Antibiotic administration neither decreases the frequency of symptomatic infection nor prevents further episodes of asymptomatic bacteriuria. Drug pressure could select MDR microorganisms.

Symptomatic bacteriuria needs withdrawal or replacement of the urinary catheter before initiating antibiotics [226]. To choose an empirical treatment, underlying conditions and the local epidemiology should be considered (risk of MDR). Carbapenems should be used in patients with high-risk Multi-Drug Resistant empirical treatment. It is important not to recommend or administer empirical antimicrobial treatment where antibiotics have more than 20% of resistant strains for non-complicated UTIs or 10% for complicated ones (Ex.: Quinolones). Treatment must be adjusted once an antimicrobial susceptibility report is available. Other antimicrobial agents are used in accordance with the aetiological agent involved (yeasts or other bacterial species). Fluconazole is the first-line antifungal agent recommended. Amphotericin B is to be used only when fluconazole resistance is suspected. The optimal treatment duration has been classically 14 days, but this can be shortened up to 5 days if there is an adequate clinical response. Follow-up urine cultures are not needed except if there is no clinical improvement 72 hours after the treatment is started.

MDR microorganisms have emerged as a potential threat to infection control. Piperacillin/tazobactam is not recommended in monotherapy as empirical treatment of CAUTI if Multi-Drug Resistant microorganism is suspected. Carbapenems can be used in monotherapy although higher dose regimens have fosfomycin [227]. Carbapenems with β-lactams/β-lactamase inhibitor combinations (BLBIC) for treatment of bacteremia due to ESBL infections. *E. coli* had no significant differences in urinary bacteremia or mortality when carbapenems with BLBIC was administered as definitive or empirical treatment. For the treatment of carbapenemases (CBP) Enterobacteriaceae; [228] *Klebsiella pneumonia*, combination therapy with at least two drugs displaying *in vitro* activity against the isolate is recommended. Combinations that included meropenem were associated with significantly higher survival rates when the meropenem MIC was $\leq$8 mg/L. Thus, for the treatment of UTI caused by MDR microorganisms, either monotherapy or bi-therapy should be decided considering the severity of infection, severity of underlying conditions, MIC values, and clinical response. Monotherapy can safely be used when no severity of signs is present. Quinolones and cotrimoxazole can be used safely as a definitive treatment only if MIC is optimal. New drugs like ceftazidime/avibactam and ceftolozane/tazobactam need further studies.

11. Conclusion

The chapter analyzes various aspects from causation to prevention and treatment of CAUTI with detailed literature for each factor involved. It addresses the various views of different researchers on each of the subtopic of catheterization keeping the cost factor also.

The final conclusion is that catheterization is inevitable but used only when it is needed. While using an appropriate method of catheterization, appropriate catheter, simple procedures of asepsis, and keeping it *in situ* only till the period that is needed are to be kept in mind. If an intermittent catheterization is needed, it should be accepted as the procedure that is needed for that particular patient (patient-centric). To keep patient care as an important priority, the HAI surveillance program is to be adopted by the hospital and carried out regularly and reviewed periodically. Appropriate corrective measures are required to prevent HAI in general and CAUTI in particular.

Acknowledgements

The author wishes to thank the Management of PESIMSR, Kuppam, Andhra Pradesh. India for their support and encouragement to bring out this chapter. The author is also thankful to Dr. Guru Vijay Kumar, Senior Resident, Community Medicine department, PESIMSR, Kuppam, AP for helping in editing the manuscript.

Conflict of interest

There is no conflict of interest in bringing out this chapter.

Author details

Chandrasekhar Nagaraj
Department of Microbiology, PESIMSR, Kuppam, Andhra Pradesh, India

*Address all correspondence to: malarianag@gmail.com

References

[1] Stamm WE, Norrby SR. Urinary tract infections: Disease panorama and challenges. The Journal of Infectious Diseases. 2001;**183**(Suppl. 1):S1-S4 11171002]

[2] Schappert SM, Rechtsteiner EA. Ambulatory medical care utilization estimates for 2007. Vital and Health Statistics. 2011;**13**:1-38

[3] Foxman B. Urinary tract infection syndromes: Occurrence, recurrence, bacteriology, risk factors, and disease burden. Infectious Disease Clinics of North America. 2014;**28**:1-13

[4] Foxman B. The epidemiology of urinary tract infection. Nature Reviews. Urology. 2010;7:653-660

[5] Hooton TM. Uncomplicated urinary tract infection. New England Journal of Medicine. 2012;**366**:1028-1037

[6] Nielubowicz GR, Mobley HL. Host–pathogen interactions in urinary tract infection. Nature Reviews. Urology. 2010;7:430-441

[7] Hannan TJ et al. Host–pathogen checkpoints and population bottlenecks in persistent and intracellular uropathogenic Escherichia coli bladder infection. FEMS Microbiology Reviews. 2012;**36**:616-648

[8] Lichtenberger P, Hooton TM. Complicated urinary tract infections. Current Infectious Disease Reports 2008; 10:499–504 18945392]

[9] Levison ME, Kaye D. Treatment of complicated urinary tract infections with an emphasis on drug-resistant gram-negative uropathogens. Current Infectious Disease Reports. 2013;**15**: 109-115

[10] Lo E et al. Strategies to prevent catheter-associated urinary tract infections in acute care hospitals: 2014 update. Infection Control and Hospital Epidemiology. 2014;**35**:464-479

[11] Flores-Mireles AL et al. Urinary tract infections: Epidemiology, mechanisms of infection and treatment options. Nature Reviews. Microbiology. 2015;**13**(5): 269-284

[12] Kline KA, Schwartz DJ, Lewis WG, Hultgren SJ, Lewis AL. Immune activation and suppression by group B Streptococcus in a murine model of urinary tract infection. Infection and Immunity. 2011;**79**:3588-3595

[13] Ronald A. The etiology of urinary tract infection: Traditional and emerging pathogens. The American Journal of Medicine. 2002;**113**(Suppl. 1A):14S-19S

[14] Fisher JF, Kavanagh K, Sobel JD, Kauffman CA, Newman C. A Candida urinary tract infection: Pathogenesis. Clinical Infectious Diseases. 2011;**52** (Suppl. 6):S437-S451

[15] Chen YH, Ko WC, Hsueh PR. Emerging resistance problems and future perspectives in pharmacotherapy for complicated urinary tract infections. Expert Opinion on Pharmacotherapy. 2013;**14**:587-596

[16] Jacobsen SM, Stickler DJ, Mobley HL, Shirtliff ME. Complicated catheter-associated urinary tract infections due to Escherichia coli and Proteus mirabilis. Clinical Microbiology Reviews. 2008;**21**:26-59

[17] Collins AS. Preventing health care-associated infections. In: Hughes RG, editor. Patient Safety and Quality: An

Evidence-Based Handbook for Nurses. Rockville (MD): Agency for Healthcare Research and Quality (US); 2008

[18] Revelas A. Healthcare - associated infections: A public health problem. Nigerian Medical Journal. 2012;**53**(2): 59-64

[19] Brennan TA, Leape LL, Laird NM, et al. Incidence of adverse events and negligence in hospitalized patients: Results of the Harvard medical practice study I. The New England Journal of Medicine. 1991;**324**(6):370-376

[20] Leape LL, Brennan TA, Laird N, et al. The nature of adverse events in hospitalized patients: Results from the Harvard medical practice study II. The New England Journal of Medicine. 1991; **324**(6):377-384

[21] Garrouste-Orgeas M, Philippart F, Bruel C, Max A, Lau N, Misset B. Overview of medical errors and adverse events. Annals of Intensive Care. 2012; **2**(1):2

[22] Parameswaran Nair N, Chalmers L, Peterson GM, Bereznicki BJ, Castelino RL, Bereznicki LR. Hospitalization in older patients due to adverse drug reactions –the need for a prediction tool. Clinical Interventions in Aging. 2016;**11**:497-505

[23] Desikan R, Krauss MJ, Dunagan WC, et al. Reporting of adverse drug events: examination of a hospital incident reporting system. In: Henriksen K, Battles JB, Marks ES, et al., editors. Advances in Patient Safety: From Research to Implementation (Volume 1: Research Findings). Rockville (MD): Agency for Healthcare Research and Quality (US); 2005

[24] Klevens RM, Edwards JR, Richards CL Jr, Horan TC, Gaynes RP, Pollock DA, et al. Estimating health care-associated infections and deaths in U.S. hospitals, 2002. Public Health Reports. 2007;**122**:160-166

[25] Agency for Healthcare Research and Quality [webpage on the Internet] Patient safety primers: Healthcare-associated infections. 2012

[26] Danasekaran R, Mani G, Annadurai K. Prevention of healthcare-associated infections: Protecting patients, saving lives. International Journal of Community Medical Public Health. 2014;**1**(1):67-68

[27] World Alliance for Patient Safety [webpage on the Internet] The Global Patient Safety Challenge 2005–2006 “Clean Care is Safer Care.”. Geneva: WHO; 2005

[28] Vincent J-L. Nosocomial infections in adult intensive-care units. Lancet. 2003;**361**(9374):2068-2077

[29] Nuvials X, Palomar M, Alvarez-Lerma F, et al. Health-care associated infections. Patient characteristics and influence on the clinical outcome of patients admitted to ICU. Intensive Care Medical Experiment. 2015;**3**(Suppl. 1):A82

[30] Johnson NB, Hayes LD, Brown K, Hoo EC, Ethier KA. Centres for Disease Control and Prevention (CDC). CDC National Health Report: Leading causes of morbidity and mortality and associated behavioral risk and protective factors-United States, 2005-2013. MMWR Suppl.ements. 2014;**63**(4):3-27

[31] McDermid RC, Stelfox HT, Bagshaw SM. Frailty in the critically ill: A novel concept. Critical Care. 2011; **15**(1):301

[32] Chernow B. Variables affecting outcome in critically ill patients. Chest. 1999;**115**(Suppl. 5):S71-S76

[33] Noakes TD, Borresen J, Hew-Butler T, Lambert MI, Jordaan E. Semmelweis and the aetiology of puerperal sepsis 160 years on: An historical review. Epidemiology and Infection. 2008; **136**(1):1-9

[34] Sydnor ERM, Perl TM. Hospital epidemiology and Infection Control in acute-care settings. Clinical Microbiology Reviews. 2011;**24**(1): 141-173

[35] In: The 2021 National and State HAI Progress Report. https://www.cdc.gov/hai/data/portal/progress-report.html

[36] Guide to the SIR Updated April 2022 (In: The NHSN Standard Infection Ratio (SIR) – CDC), pp 1–50

[37] A Guide to the SUR Updated April 2022 (In: The NHSN Standard Utilization Ratio (SUR) – CDC), pp 1-28

[38] Chenoweth CE, Gould CV, Saint S. Diagnosis, management, and prevention of catheter-associated urinary tract infections. Infectious Disease Clinics of North America. 2014;**28**:105-119

[39] Al-Tafiq JA, Tambyah PA. Healthcare associated infections (HAI) perspectives. Journal of Infection and Public Health. 2014;7:339-344

[40] Obaid NA. Preventive measures and Management of Catheter-Associated Urinary Tract Infection in adult Intensive Care Units in Saudi Arabia. Journal of Epidemiology Global Health. 2021;**11**:164-168

[41] Rosenthal VD. Device-associated nosocomial infections in 55 intensive care units of 8 developing countries. Annals of Internal Medicine. 2006;**145**: 582-591

[42] Storme O, Tiran Saucedo J, Garcia-Mora A, Dehesa-Davila M, Naber KG. Risk factors and predisposing conditions for urinary tract infection. Therapeutic Advances in Urology. 2019;**11**:19-28

[43] Guneysel O, Onur O, Erdede M, Denizbasi A. Trimethoprim / sulfamethoxazole resistance in urinary tract infections. The Journal of Emergency Medicine. 2009;**36**:338-341

[44] Bagchi I, Jaitly NK, Thombare V. Microbiological evaluation of catheter associated urinary tract infection in a tertiary care hospital. People's Journal of Scientific Research. 2015;**8**:23-29

[45] Zahran F. Catheter associated Urinary tract Infection (Cauti) in MedicalWard, and Icu Kfhh during year 2017. International Journal of Advanced Research. 2018;**6**:997-1011

[46] Dalen DM, Zvonar RK, Jessamine PG. An evaluation of the management of asymptomatic catheter-associated bacteriuria and candiduria at the Ottawa Hospital. Canadian Journal of Infectious Diseases Medical Microbiology. 2005;**16**:166-170

[47] Martin CM, Bookrajian EN. Bacteruria prevention after indwelling urinary catheterization. Archives of Internal Medicine. 1962:703-711

[48] Saint S. Clinical and economic consequences of nosocomial catheter related bacteriuria. Journal of Infectious Control. 2000;**28**:68-75

[49] Paget G, Naicker S, Perovic O. Guidelines for the management of nosocomial urinary tract infections. The South Africa Journal of Epidemiological Infection. 2005;**20**(2):58-60

[50] Saint S, Chenoweth CE. Biofilms and catheter-associated urinary tract

infections. Infectious Disease Clinics of North America. 2003;**17**(2):411-432

[51] Saint S, Wiese J, Amory JK, Bernstein ML, Patel UD, Zemencuk JK, et al. Are physicians aware of which of their patients have indwelling urinary catheters? The American Journal of Medicine. 2000;**109**(6):476-480

[52] Humphreys H, Newcombe RG, Enstone J, Smyth ET, McIlvenny G, Fitzpatrick F, et al. Four country healthcare associated infection prevalence survey 2006: Risk factor analysis. The Journal of Hospital Infection. 2008;**69**(3):249-257

[53] Garibaldi RA, Burke JP, Dickman ML, Smith CB. Factors predisposing to bacteriuria during indwelling urethral catheterization. The New England Journal of Medicine. 1974; **291**(5):215-219

[54] Haley RW, Hooton TM, Culver DH, Stanley RC, Emori TG, Hardison CD, et al. Nosocomial infections in U.S. hospitals, 1975-1976: Estimated frequency by selected characteristics of patients. The American Journal of Medicine. 1981; **70**(4):947-959

[55] Tambyah PA, Maki DG. Catheter-associated urinary tract infection is rarely symptomatic: A prospective study of 1,497 catheterized patients. Archives of Internal Medicine. 2000;**160**(5): 678-682

[56] Scottish Intercollegiate Guideline Network. Management of Suspected Bacterial Urinary Tract Infection in Adults. A National Clinical Guideline; Edinburgh: SIGN; 2006

[57] Elvy J, Colville A. Catheter-associated urinary tract infection: What is it, what causes it and how can we prevent it? Journal of Infection Prevention. 2009;**10**(2):36-41

[58] Maki DG, Tambyah PA. Engineering out the risk for infection with urinary catheters. Emerging Infectious Diseases. 2001;7(2):342-347

[59] Tissot E, Limat S, Cornette C, Capellier G. Risk factors for catheter-associated bacteriuria in a medical intensive care unit. European Journal of Clinical Microbiology & Infectious Diseases. 2001;**20**(4):260-262

[60] Tambyah PA, Halvorson KT, Maki DG. A prospective study of pathogenesis of catheter-associated urinary tract infections. Mayo Clinic Proceedings. 1999;**74**(2):131-136

[61] Platt R, Polk BF, Murdock B, Rosner B. Risk factors for nosocomial urinary tract infection. American Journal of Epidemiology. 1986;**124**(6):977-985

[62] Shapiro M, Simchen E, Izraeli S, Sacks TG. A multivariate analysis of risk factors for acquiring bacteriuria in patients with indwelling urinary catheters for longer than 24 hours. Infection Control. 1984;**5**(11):525-532

[63] Coello R, Charlett A, Ward V, Wilson J, Pearson A, Sedgwick J, et al. Device-related sources of bacteraemia in English hospitals–opportunities for the prevention of hospital-acquired bacteraemia. Journal of Hospital Infection. 2003 Jan;**53**(1):46-57

[64] Holroyd-Leduc JM, Sen S, Bertenthal D, Sands LP, Palmer RM, Kresevic DM, et al. The relationship of indwelling urinary catheters to death, length of hospital stay, functional decline, and nursing home admission in hospitalized older medical patients. Journal of the American Geriatrics Society. 2007 Feb;**55**(2):227-233

[65] Ovbiagele B, Hills N, Saver J, Claiborne JS. Frequency of determinates of pneumonia and Urinary tract Infection. Journal of Stroke and Cerebrovascular Diseases. 2006;**15**(5): 209-213

[66] Oza A, Cunney R. Enhanced bacteraemia surveillance in Ireland 2004 and 2005. Epi-Insight 7. 2006

[67] Andreu A, Cacho J, Coira A, Lepe JA. Microbiological diagnosis of urinary tract infections. Enfermedades Infecciosas y Microbiología Clínica. 2011;**29**:52-57

[68] Horcajada JP, Shaw E, Padilla B, Pintado V, Calbo E, Benito N, et al. Healthcare-associated, community-acquired and hospital-acquired bacteraemic urinary tract infections in hospitalized patients: A prospective multicentre cohort study in the era of antimicrobial resistance. Clinical Microbiology and Infection. 2013;**19**: 962-968

[69] Nicolle LE. The chronic indwelling catheter and urinary infection in long-term-care facility residents. Infection Control and Hospital Epidemiology. 2001 May;**22**(5):316-321

[70] Nguyen-Van-Tam SE, Nguyen-Van-Tam JS, Myint S, Pearson JC. Risk factors for hospital-acquired urinary tract infection in a large English teaching hospital: A case-control study. Infection. 1999 May;**27**(3):192-197

[71] Graves N, Tong E, Morton AP, Halton K, Curtis M, Lairson D, et al. Factors associated with health care-acquired urinary tract infection. American Journal of Infection Control. 2007;**35**(6):387-392

[72] Govindarajan DK, Kandaswamy K. Virulence factors of uropathogens and their role in host pathogen interactions. The Cell Surface. 2022;**8**:1-12

[73] Rezatofighi SE, Mirzarazi M. Virulence genes and phylogenetic groups of uropathogenic *Escherichia coli* isolates from patients with urinary tract infection and uninfected control subjects: a case control study. BMC Infectious Diseases. 2021;**21**:1-11

[74] Saint S, Lipsky B. Preventing catheter-related bacteriuria: Should we? Can we? How? Archives of Internal Medicine. 1999;**159**(8):800-808

[75] Gould CV, Umscheid CA, Agarwai RK, Kuntz G, Pesueo DA. Guideline for Prevention of Catheter Associated Urinary Tract Infections. 2010;**31**: 319-326

[76] Tenke P, Kovacs B, Bjerldund-Johansen T, Matsumoto T, Tambyah P, Naber K. European and Asian guidelines on management and prevention of catheter-associated urinary tract infections. International Journal of Antimicrobial Agents. 2007;**31**(S1):68-78

[77] Hooton TM, Bradley SF, Cardenas DD, Colgan R, Geerlings SE, Rice JC, et al. Diagnosis, prevention, and treatment of catheter-associated urinary tract infection in adults: 2009 International Clinical Practice Guidelines from the Infectious Diseases Society of America. Clinical Infectious Diseases. 2010;**50**(5):625-663

[78] Gokula RR, Hickner JA, Smith MA. Inappropriate use of urinary catheters in elderly patients at a Midwestern community teaching hospital. American Journal of Infection Control. 2004;**32**(4): 196-199

[79] Jain P, Parada JP, David A, Smith LG. Overuse of the indwelling

urinary tract catheter in hospitalized medical patients. Archives of Internal Medicine. 1995;**155**(13):1425-1429

[80] Munasinghe RL, Yazdani H, Siddique M, Hafeez W. Appropriateness of use of indwelling urinary catheters in patients admitted to the medical service. Infection Control and Hospital Epidemiology. 2001;**22**(10):647-649

[81] Wong ES. Guideline for prevention of catheter-associated urinary tract infections. American Journal of Infection Control. 1983;**11**(1):28-36

[82] Pratt RJ et al. Epic 2: National evidence-based guidelines for preventing healthcare associated infections in NHS hospitals in England. The Journal of Hospital Infection. 2007;**6** (Suppl. 1):S1-S64

[83] Pellowe CM, Pratt RJ, Harper P, Loveday HP, Robinson N, Jones SR, et al. Evidence-based guidelines for preventing healthcare-associated infections in primary and community care in England. The Journal of Hospital Infection. 2003;**55**(Suppl. 2):S2-S127

[84] Matlow AG, Wray RD, Cox PH. Nosocomial urinary tract infections in a paediatric intensive care unit: A follow-up after 10 years. Pediatric Critical Care Medicine. 2003;**4**(1):74-77

[85] Talja M, Korpela A, Jarvi K. Comparison of urethral reaction to full silicone, hydrogen-coated and siliconised latex catheters. British Journal of Urology. 1990;**66**(6):652-657

[86] Robertson GS, Everitt N, Burton PR, Flynn JT. Effect of catheter material on the incidence of urethral strictures. British Journal of Urology. 1991;**68**(6): 612-617

[87] Saint S, Kaufman SR, Rogers MA, Baker PD, Boyko EJ, Lipsky BA. Risk factors for nosocomial urinary tract related bacteremia: A case-control study. American Journal of Infection Control. 2006;**34**(7):401-407

[88] Lopez-Lopez G, Pascual A, Martinez-Martinez L, Perea EJ. Effect of siliconized latex urinary catheter on bacterial adherence and human neutrophil activity. Diagnostic Microbiology and Infectious Disease. 1991;**14**(1):1-6

[89] Moore KN, Fader M, Getliffe K. Long-term bladder management by intermittent catheterization in adults and children. Cochrane Database of Systematic Reviews. 2007;**4**:CD006008

[90] Chai T, Chung AK, Belville WD, Faerber GJ. Compliance and complications of clean intermittent catheterization in the spinal cord injured patient. Paraplegia. 1995 Mar;**33**(3):161-163

[91] Schumm K, Lam TBL. Types of urethral catheters for management of short-term voiding problems in hospitalized adults: A systematic review (structured abstract). Cochrane Database of Abstracts of Reviews of Effects. 2008;**2008**:1-37

[92] Chaiban G, Hanna H, Dvorak T, Raad I. A rapid method of impregnating endotracheal tubes and urinary catheters with gendine: A novel antiseptic agent. Journal of Antimicrobial Chemotherapy. 2000;**55**(1):51-56

[93] Cho YW, Park JH, Kim SH, Cho YH, Choi JM, Shin HJ, et al. Gentamicin-releasing urethral catheter for short-term catheterization. Journal of Biomaterials Science, Polymer Edition. 2003;**14**(9): 963-972

[94] Gentry H, Cope S. Using silver to reduce catheter associated urinary tract

infections. Nursing Standard. 2005; **19**(50):51-54

[95] Johnson JR, Kuskowski MA, Wilt TJ. Systematic review: Antimicrobial urinary catheters to prevent catheter associated urinary tract infection in hospitalized patients. Annals of Internal Medicine. 2006;**144**(2): 116-127

[96] Karchmer TB, Giannetta ET, Muto CA, Strain BA, Farr BM. A randomized crossover study of silver-coated urinary catheters in hospitalized patients. Archives of Internal Medicine. 2000;**160**(3):3294-3298

[97] Lai KK. Use of silver-hydrogel urinary catheters on the incidence of catheter associated urinary tract infections in hospitalized patients. American Journal of Infection Control. 2002;**30**(4):221-225

[98] Madeo M, Davies D, Johnson G, Owen E, Wadsworth P, Mmiin CR. The impact of using silver alloy urinary catheters in reducing the incidence of urinary tract infections in the critical care setting. British Journal of Infection Control. 2005;**5**(1):21-24

[99] Newton T, Still JM, Law EA. Comparison of the effect of early insertion of standard latex and silver impregnated latex Foley catheters on urinary tract infections in bum patients. Infection Control and Hospital Epidemiology. 2002;**23**(4): 217-218

[100] Niel-Weise BS, Arend SM, van den Broek PJ. Is there evidence for recommending silver-coated urinary catheters in guidelines? Journal of Hospital Infection. 2002;**52**(2):81-87

[101] Rupp ME, Fitzgerald T, Marion N, Helget V, Puumala S, Anderson JR, et al. Effect of silver-coated urinary catheters: Efficacy, cost-effectiveness, and antimicrobial resistance. American Journal of Infection Control. 2004;**32**(8): 445-450

[102] Saint S, Elmore J, Sullivan S. The efficacy of silver alloy-coated urinary catheters in preventing urinary tract infection: A meta-analysis. Journal of Urology. 1998; **162**(1):283-284

[103] Thibon P, Le Coutour X, Leroyer R, Fabry J. Randomized multi-Centre trial of the effects of a catheter coated with hydrogel and silver salts on the incidence of hospital acquired urinary tract infections. Journal of Hospital Infection. 2000;**45**(2):117-124

[104] Drekonja DM, Kuskowski MA, Wilt TJ, Johnson JR. Antimicrobial urinary catheters: A systematic review. Expert Review Medical Devices. 2008; **5**(4):495-506

[105] Dieckhaus KD, Garibaldi RA. Prevention of catheter-associated urinary tract infections. In: Abrutytn E, Goldman DA, Scheckler WE, editors. Saunders Infection Control Reference Service. Philadelphia: Saunders Co; 1998. pp. 167-174

[106] Roe BH, Brocklehurst JC. Study of patients with indwelling catheters. Journal of Advanced Nursing. 1987 Nov; **12**(6):713-718

[107] National Patient Safety Agency. Female urinary catheters causing trauma to adult males. 2009. Ref Type: Online Source

[108] Newman DK. Internal and external urinary catheters: A primer for clinical practice. Ostomy/Wound Management. 2008 Dec;**54**(12):18-35

[109] Nickel JC, Feero P, Costerton JW, Wilson E. Incidence and importance of bacteriuria in postoperative, short-term urinary catheterization. Canadian Journal of Surgery. 1989 Mar;**32**(2): 131-132

[110] Pratt RJ, Pellowe CM, Wilson JA, Loveday HP, Harper PJ, Jones SR, et al. epic2: National evidence-based guidelines for preventing healthcare-associated infections in NHS hospitals in England. Journal of Hospital Infection. 2007;**65**(Suppl. 1):S1-S64

[111] Jahn P, Beutner K, Langer G. Types of indwelling urinary catheters for long-term bladder drainage in adults. Cochrane Database Syst Rev. 2012 Oct 17;**10**:CD004997. DOI: 10.1002/14651858.CD004997. pub3. PMID: 23076911 Review

[112] Thibon P, Le C, Leroyer R, Fabry J. Randomized multi-Centre trial of the effects of a catheter coated with hydrogel and silver salts on the incidence of hospital-acquired urinary tract infections. The Journal of Hospital Infection. 2000 Jun;**45**(2):117-124

[113] Gaonkar TA, Sampath LA, Modak SM. Evaluation of the antimicrobial efficacy of urinary catheters impregnated with antiseptics in an in vitro urinary tract model. Infection Control and Hospital Epidemiology. 2003 Jul;**24**(7):506-513

[114] Darouiche RO, Smith JA Jr, Hanna H, Dhabuwala CB, Steiner MS, Babaian RJ, et al. Efficacy of antimicrobial impregnated bladder catheters in reducing catheter-associated bacteriuria: A prospective, randomized, multicentre clinical trial. Urology. 1999 Dec;**54**(6):976-981

[115] Al-Habdan I, Sadat-Ali M, Corea JR, Al-Othman A, Kamal BA, Shriyan DS. Assessment of nosocomial urinary tract infections in orthopaedic patients: A prospective and comparative study using two different catheters. International Surgery. 2003 Jul;**88**(3):152-154

[116] Brosnahan J, Jull A, Tracy C. Types of urethral catheters for management of short-term voiding problems in hospitalised adults. Cochrane Database of Systematic Reviews. 2002;**1**: CD004013

[117] Pratt RJ, Pellowe C, Loveday HP, Robinson N, Smith GW, Barrett S, et al. The epic project: Developing national evidence based guidelines for preventing hospital-acquired infections. Phase 1: Guidelines for preventing hospital-acquired infections. Journal of Hospital Infection. 2022;**47**(Suppl. 1):S3-S82

[118] Riley DK, Classen DC, Stevens LE, Burke JP. A large randomized clinical trial of a silver-impregnated urinary catheter: Lack of efficacy and staphylococcal super infection. The American Journal of Medicine. 1995; **98**(4):349-356

[119] Health Information and Quality Authority. National Standards for the Prevention and Control of Healthcare Associated Infection. Dublin: Heath Information and Quality Authority; 2009

[120] Magnall J, Watterson L. Principles of aseptic technique in urinary catheterization. Nursing Standard. 2006; **21**(8):49-56

[121] Siegel JD, Rhinehart E, Jackson M, Chiarello L. 2007 guideline for isolation precautions: Preventing transmission of infectious agents in health care settings. American Journal of Infection Control. 2007;**35**(10 Suppl. 2):S65-S164

[122] Desautels RE, Walter CW, Graves RC, Harrison JH. Technical

advances in the prevention of urinary tract infection. The Journal of Urology. 1962;**87**:487-490

[123] Kass EH, Schneiderman LJ. Entry of bacteria into the urinary tracts of patients with inlying catheters. The New England Journal of Medicine. 1957; **256**(12):556-557

[124] Kunin CM. Urinary Tract Infections: Detection, Prevention and Management. Baltimore: Williams and Wilkins; 1997

[125] Kunin CM, McCormack RC. Prevention of catheter-induced urinary-tract infections by sterile closed drainage. The New England Journal of Medicine. 1966;**274**(21):1155-1161

[126] Rowley S. Aseptic on-touch technique. Nursing Times. 2001;**97**(7):6

[127] SARI Infection Control Sub-committee. Health Protection Surveillance Centre. Dublin. Guidelines for hand hygiene in Irish healthcare settings. 2005

[128] World Health Organisation. Guidelines on Hand Hygiene in Healthcare. 2009. Ref Type: Online Source

[129] Warren JW. Catheter-associated urinary tract infections. Infectious Disease Clinics of North America. 1997; **11**(3):609-622

[130] Association for Continence Advice. Notes on Good Practice. 2007. http://www.notesongoodpractice.co.uk/

[131] Dunn S. Management of short-term indwelling urethral catheters to prevent urinary tract infections. A systematic review. 2000. The Joanna Briggs Institute for Evidence Based Nursing and Midwifery.

[132] Page LC, Conroy-Hiller T, T. Florence Z. Management of short-term indwelling urethral catheters to prevent urinary tract infections. International Journal of Evidence-Based Healthcare. 2004;**2**(8):271-291

[133] Australian Guidelines for the Prevention and Control of Infection in Healthcare Australian Guidelines for the Prevention and Control of Infection in Healthcare. National Health and Medical Research Council May 2019. 2020. Website Reference number CD34 ISBN online 978-1-86496-028-0

[134] Panknin HT, Althaus P. Guidelines for preventing infections associated with the insertion and maintenance of short-term indwelling urethral catheters in acute care. The Journal of Hospital Infection. 2001;**49**(2):146-147

[135] National Collaborating Centre for Women's and Children's Health. Prevention and Treatment of Surgical Site Infection. London: RCOG Press; 2008

[136] Department of Health and Aging Austrialian Government. Infection control guidelines for the prevention of transmission of infectious diseases in the healthcare setting. 2004.

[137] Dmm S, Pretty L, Reid H, Evans D. Management of Short Term Indwelling Urethral Catheters to Prevent Urinary Tract Infections. A Systematic Review. Australia: The Joanna Briggs Institute for Evidence Based Nursing and Midwifery; 2000

[138] Ward V, Wilson J, Taylor L, Cookson B, Glynn A. Preventing Hospital-Acquired Infection: Clinical Guidelines. London: Public Health Laboratory Service; 1997

[139] Dieckhaus KD, Garibaldi RA. Prevention of catheter-associated

urinary tract infections. In: Abmtytn E, Goldmann DA, Scheckler WE, editors. Saunders Infection Control Reference Service. Philadelphia: Saunders; 1998. pp. 169-174

[140] Kunin CM. Urinary Tract Infections: Detection, Prevention and Management. 5th ed. Baltimore: Williams & Wilkins; 1997. pp. 228-229

[141] Stamm WE. Catheter-associated urinary tract infections: Epidemiology, pathogenesis, and prevention. American Journal of Medicine. 1991;**91**(Suppl. 3B): 65-71

[142] Stamm WE. Urinary tract infections. In: Bennett JV, Brachman PS, editors. Hospital Infection. 4th ed. Philadelphia: Lippincott-Raven; 1998. pp. 477-485

[143] Carpeti EA, Andrews SM, Bentley PG. Randomized study of sterile versus non-sterile urethral catheterization. Annals of the Royal College of Surgeons of England. 1996; 7(1):59-60

[144] Bardsley A. Use of lubricant gels in urinary catheterization. Nursing Standard. 2005;**20**(8):41-46

[145] Dougherty L, Lister S. The Royal Marsden Hospital Manual of Clinical Nursing Procedures. 7th ed. London: Wiley-Blackwell; 2008

[146] Burke JP, Riley DK. Nosocomial urinary tract infection. In: Mayhall CG, editor. Hospital Epidemiology and Infection Control. Philadelphia: Lippincott Williams & Wilkins; 1996. pp. 139-153

[147] Gardam MA, Amihod B, Orenstein P, Consolacion N, Miller MA. Ovemtilization of indwelling catheters and the development of nosocomial urinary tract infection. Clinical Peljormance Quality Health Care. 1998; **6**(3):99-102

[148] Niel-Weise BS, van den Broeck PJ. Antibiotic policies for short-term catheter bladder drainage in adults. Cochrane Database of Systematic Reviews. 2005;**3**:CD005428

[149] Saint S, Veenstra D, Sullivan S, Chenoweth C, Fendrick A. The potential clinical and economic benefits of silver alloy urinary catheters in preventing urinary tract infection. Archives of Internal Medicine. 2000;**160**(17): 2670-2675

[150] Van den Eijkel E, Griffiths P. Catheter valves for indwelling urinary catheters: A systematic review. British Journal of Community Nursing. 2006; **11**(3):111-114

[151] Burke JP, Garibaldi RA, Britt MR, Jacobson JA, Conti M, Alling DW. Prevention of catheter-associated urinary tract infections: Efficacy of daily meatal care regimens. American Journal of Medicine. 1981;**70**(3):655-658

[152] Burke JP, Jacobson JA, Garibaldi RA, Conti MT, Alling DW. Evaluation of daily meatal care with poly-antibiotic ointment in prevention of urinary catheter- associated bacteriuria. Journal of Urology. 1983; **129**(2):331-334

[153] Classen DC, Larsen RA, Burke JP, Alling DW, Stevens LE. Daily meatal care for prevention of catheter-associated bacteriuria: Results using frequent applications of polyantibiotic cream. Infection Control and Hospital Epidemiology. 1991;**12**(3):157-162

[154] Crouzet J, Bertrand X, Venier AG, Badoz M, Husson C, Talon D. Control of

the duration of urinary catheterization: Impact on catheter associated urinary tract infection. The Journal of Hospital Infection. 2007;**67**(3):253-257

[155] Griffiths R, Fernandez R. Strategies for the removal of short-term indwelling urethral catheters in adults. Cochrane Database of Systematic Reviews. 2007;**2**: CD004011. DOI: 10.1002/14651858. CD00401l.pub3

[156] Phipps S, Lim YN, McClinton S, Barry C, Rane A, N'Dow J. Short term urinary catheter policies following urogenital surgery in adults. Cochrane Database of Systematic Reviews. 2006;**2**: CD004374. DOI: 10.10002/14651858. CD004374.pub2

[157] Apisarnthanarak A, Thongphubeth K, Sirinvaravong S, Kitkangvan D, Yuekyen C, Warachan B, et al. Effectiveness of multifaceted hospital wide quality improvement programs featuring an intervention to remove unnecessary urinary catheters at a tertiary care center in Thailand. Infection Control and Hospital Epidemiology. 2007;**28**(7):791-798

[158] Nicolle LE. Catheter-related urinary tract infection. Drugs & Aging. 2005; **22**(8):627-639

[159] Agodi A, Barchitta M, Anzaldi A, Marchese F, Bonaccorsi A, Motta M. Active surveillance of nosocomial infections in urologic patients. European Urology. 2009;**51**(1):247-254

[160] Smith PW, Bennett G, Bradley S, Drinka P, Lautenbach E, Marx J, et al. SHEA/APIC guideline: Infection prevention and control in the long-term care facility. American Journal of Infection Control. 2008 Sep;**36**(7):504-535

[161] Consortium for Spinal Cord Medicine. Bladder management in adults with spinal cord injury: A clinical practice guideline for health-care providers. The Journal of Spinal Cord Medicine. 2006;**29**(5):527-573

[162] Dille CM, Kirchhoff KT. Decontamination of vinyl urinary drainage bags with bleach. Rehabilitation Nursing. 1993;**18**(5):292-295

[163] Hashisaki P, Swenson J, Mooney B, Epstein B, Bowcutt C. Decontamination of urinary bags for rehabilitation patients. Archives of Physical Medicine and Rehabilitation. 1984;**65**(8):474-476

[164] Rooney M. Impacting health care: Study of a reusable urinary drainage system. SCI Nursing. 1994;**11**(1):16-18

[165] Toughill E. Indwelling urinary catheters: Common mechanical and pathogenic problems. The American Journal of Nursing. 2005;**105**(5):35-37

[166] Wright D, Pomfret I. Urinary catheterization: The infection control aspects. Journal of Community Nursing. 2010;**23**(3):11-14

[167] Platt R, Polk BF, Murdock B, Rosner B. Reduction of mortality associated with nosocomial urinary tract infection. Lancet. 1983;**1**(8330): 893-897

[168] DeGroot-Kosolcharoen J, Guse R, Jones JM. Evaluation of a urinary catheter with a preconnected closed drainage bag. Infection Control and Hospital Epidemiology. 1988;**9**(2):72-76

[169] Leone M, Garnier F, Antonini F, Bimar MC, Albanese J, Martin C. Comparison of effectiveness of two urinary drainage systems in intensive care unit: A prospective, randomized clinical trial. Intensive Care Medicine. 2003;**29**(3):410-413

[170] Newman DK. The indwelling urinary catheter: Principles for best practice. Journal of Wound, Ostomy, and Continence Nursing. 2007;**34**(6): 655-661

[171] McCann M, Hennigan M, Hawshaw S. Nurse's knowledge of infection control measures preventing urinary tract infections in catheterised patients. In: Proceedings of the 26th International Nursing and Midwifery Research Conference. Dublin; 2007

[172] Addison R. Catheter valves: A special focus on the bard Flip-Flo catheter. The British Journal of Nursing. 1999;**8**(9):576-580

[173] Doherty W. The Sims Portex catheter valve: An alternative to the leg bag. The British Journal of Nursing. 1999;**8**(7):459-462

[174] Fader M, Pettersson L, Brooks R, Dean G, Wells M, Cottenden A, et al. A multicentre comparative evaluation of catheter valves. The British Journal of Nursing. 1997;**6**(7):359

[175] Pomfret I. Catheter care in the community. Nursing Standard. 2000; **14**(27):46-51

[176] Pettersson L, Fader M. Choosing a catheter valve that suits the patient. Community Nurse. 1997 May;**3**(4):9

[177] Gray ML. Securing the indwelling catheter. The American Journal of Nursing. 2008;**108**(12):44-50

[178] Senese V, Hendricks B, Morrison M, Harris J. Clinical practice guidelines: Care of the patient with an indwelling catheter. Urologic Nursing. 2006;**26**(1): 80-81

[179] Gray M. What nursing interventions reduce the risk of symptomatic urinary tract infection in the patient with an indwelling catheter? Journal of Wound, Ostomy, and Continence Nursing. 2004;**31**(1):3-13

[180] Darouiche RO, Goetz L, Kaldis T, Cerra-Stewart C, AlSharif A, Priebe M. Impact of stat lock securing device on symptomatic catheter-related urinary tract infection: A prospective, randomized, multicentre clinical trial. American Journal of Infection Control. 2006;**34**(9):555-560

[181] Pomfret IJ. Catheters: Design, selection and management. The British Journal of Nursing. 1996;**5**(4): 245-251

[182] Fraise AP, Bradley C. Ayliffe's Control of Hospital Infection - a Practical Handbook. 5th ed. London: Hodder Arnold; 2009

[183] Joanna Briggs Institute. Management of Indwelling Urethral Catheters to Prevent Urinary Tract Infection. 2000.

[184] Getliffe K. Catheter blockage in community patients. Nursing Standard. 1990;**5**(9):33-36

[185] McCarthy K, Hunter I. Importance of pH monitoring in the care of long-term catheters. The British Journal of Nursing. 2001;**10**(19):1240-1247

[186] Stephan F, Sax H, Wachsmuth M, Hoffmeyer P, Clergue F, Pittet D. Reduction of urinary tract infection and antibiotic use after surgery: A controlled, prospective, before-after intervention study. Clinical Infectious Diseases. 2006; **42**(11):1544-1551

[187] Doyle B, Mawji Z, Horgan M, Stelliman P, et al. Decreasing nosocomial urinary tract infection in a large

academic community hospital. Lippincott's Case Management. 2001; **6**(3):127-136

[188] Cornia PB, Amory JK, Fraser S, Saint S, Lipsky BA. Computer-based order entry decreases duration of indwelling urinary catheterization in hospitalized patients. The American Journal of Medicine. 2003;**114**(5): 404-407

[189] Huang WC, Wann SR, Lin SL, Kunin CM, Kung MH, Lin CH, et al. Catheter-associated urinary tract infections in intensive care units can be reduced by prompting physicians to remove unnecessary catheters. Infection Control and Hospital Epidemiology. 2004;**25**(11):974-978

[190] Saint S, Kaufman SR, Thompson M, Rogers MA, Chenoweth CE. A reminder reduces urinary catheterization in hospitalized patients. Joint Commission Journal on Quality and Patient Safety. 2005;**31**(8):455-462

[191] Topal J, Conklin S, Camp K, Morris V, Balcezak T, Herbert P. Prevention of nosocomial catheter-associated urinary tract infections through computerized feedback to physicians and a nurse-directed protocol. American Journal of Medical Quality. 2005;**20**(3):121-126

[192] Meddings J, Rogers MA, Macy M, Saint S. Systematic review and meta-analysis: Reminder systems to reduce catheter-associated urinary tract infections and urinary catheter use in hospitalized patients. Clinical Infectious Diseases. 2010;**51**(5):550-560

[193] Levy MM, Dellinger RP, Townsend SR, Linde-Zwirble WT, Marshall JC, Bion J, et al. The surviving Sepsis campaign: Results of an international guideline-based performance improvement program targeting severe sepsis. Intensive Care Medicine. 2010;**36**(2):222-231

[194] Mayumi T, Takada T, Hirata K, Yoshida M, Sekimoto M, Hirota M, et al. Pancreatitis bundles. Journal of Hepato-Biliary-Pancreatic Surgery. 2009;**2009**: 11

[195] Powers RJ, Wirtschafter DW. Decreasing central line associated bloodstream infection in neonatal intensive care. Clinics in Perinatology. 2010;**37**(1):247-272

[196] Rello J, Lode H, Cornaglia G, Masterton R. A European care bundle for prevention of ventilator-associated pneumonia. Intensive Care Medicine. 2010;**36**(5):773-780

[197] Venkatram S, Rachmale S, Kanna B. Study of device use adjusted rates in health care-associated infections after implementation of "bundles" in a closed-model medical intensive care unit. Journal of Critical Care. 2010;**25**(1): 174-178

[198] Wazait HD, van der Meullen J, Patel HR, Brown CT, Gadgil S, Miller RA, et al. Antibiotics on urethral catheter withdrawal: A hit and miss affair. The Journal of Hospital Infection. 2004;**58**(4):297-302

[199] Niel-Weise BS, van den Broek PJ. Urinary catheter policies for long-term bladder drainage. Cochrane Database of Systematic Reviews. 2005;**1**:CD004201

[200] Olson ES, Cookson BD. Do antimicrobials have a role in preventing septicaemia following instrumentation of the urinary tract? The Journal of Hospital Infection. 2000;**45**(2):85-97

[201] Jewes LA, Gillespie WA, Leadbetter A, Myers B, Simpson RA,

Stower MJ, et al. Bacteriuria and bacteraemia in patients with long-term indwelling catheters–a domiciliary study. Journal of Medical Microbiology. 1988;**26**(1):61-65

[202] NICE Short Clinical Guidelines Technical Team. Prophylaxis against Infective Endocarditis: Antimicrobial Prophylaxis against Infective Endocarditis in Adults and Children Undergoing Interventional Procedures. London: National Institute for Health and Clinical Excellence; 2008

[203] Gould FK, Elliott TS, Foweraker J, Fulford M, Perry JD, Roberts GJ, et al. Guidelines for the prevention of endocarditis: Report of the working Party of the British Society for antimicrobial chemotherapy. The Journal of Antimicrobial Chemotherapy. 2006;**57**(6):1035-1042

[204] Wilson W, Taubert KA, Gewitz M, Lockhart PB, Baddour LM, Levison M, et al. Prevention of infective endocarditis: Guidelines from the American Heart Association: a guideline from the American Heart Association Rheumatic Fever, Endocarditis, and Kawasaki Disease Committee, Council on Cardiovascular Disease in the Young, and the Council on Clinical Cardiology, Council on Cardiovascular Surgery and Anesthesia, and the Quality of Care and Outcomes Research Interdisciplinary Working Group. Circulation. 2007; **116**(15):1736-1754

[205] Garner JS, Jarvis WR, Emori TG, Horan TC, Hughes JM. CDC definitions for nosocomial infections, 1988. American Journal of Infection Control. 1988;**16**(3):128-140

[206] Leblebicioglu H, Esen S. Hospital-acquired urinary tract infections in Turkey: A nationwide multicentre point prevalence study. The Journal of Hospital Infection. 2003;**53**(3): 207-210

[207] Reilly J, Stewart S, Allardice GA, Noone A, Robertson C, Walker A, et al. Results from the Scottish national HAI prevalence survey. The Journal of Hospital Infection. 2008;**69**(1):62-68

[208] Lee MK, Chiu CS, Chow VC, Lam RK, Lai RW. Prevalence of hospital infection and antibiotic use at a university medical center in Hong Kong. The Journal of Hospital Infection. 2007; **65**(4):341-347

[209] Elpern EH, Killeen K, Ketchem A, Wiley A, Patel G, Lateef O. Reducing use of indwelling urinary catheters and associated urinary tract infections. American Journal of Critical Care. 2009; **18**(6):535-541

[210] Madani N, Rosenthal VD, Dendane T, Abidi K, Zeggwagh AA, Abouqal R. Health-care associated infections rates, length of stay, and bacterial resistance in an intensive care unit of Morocco: Findings of the International Nosocomial Infection Control consortium (INICC). International Archives of Medicine. 2009;**2**(1):29

[211] Rebmann T, Greene LR. Preventing catheter-associated urinary tract infections: An executive summary of the Association for Professionals in Infection Control and epidemiology, Inc, Elimination Guide. American Journal of Infectious Control. 2010;**38**(8): 644-646

[212] Rosenthal VD, Maki DG, Jamulitrat S, Medeiros EA, Todi SK, Gomez DY, et al. International Nosocomial Infection Control Consortium (INICC) report, data

summary for 2003-2008, issued June 2009. American Journal of Infectious Control. 2010;**38**(2): 95-104

[213] Weber DJ, Brown V, Huslage K, Sickbert-Bennett E, Rutala WA. Device-related infections in home health care and hospice: Infection rates, 1998-2008. Infection Control and Hospital Epidemiology. 2009;**30**(10):1022-1024

[214] Horan TC, Andrus M, Dudeck MA. CDC/NHSN surveillance definition of health care-associated infection and criteria for specific types of infections in the acute care setting. American Journal of Infection Control. 2008;**36**(5):309-332

[215] Hospital in Europe Link for Infection Control through Surveillance. Surveillance of Nosocomial Infections in Intensive Care Units - Protocol. Version 6.1. 2004

[216] Kaye D. Urinary tract infections in the elderly. Bulletin of the New York Academy of Medicine. 1980;**56**(2): 209-220

[217] Babcock HM, Zack JE, Garrison T, Trovillion E, Jones M, Fraser VJ, et al. An educational intervention to reduce ventilator-associated pneumonia in an integrated health system: A comparison of effects. Chest. 2004;**125**(6):2224-2231

[218] Warren DK, Zack JE, Mayfield JL, Chen A, Prentice D, Fraser VJ, et al. The effect of an education program on the incidence of central venous catheter-associated bloodstream infection in a medical ICU. Chest. 2004 Nov;**126**(5): 1612-1618

[219] Prout S. Development of guidelines on obtaining catheter specimens of urine utilising a closed system with an incorporated safety gaurd mechanism for needle disposal. In: Proceedings of the 28th International Nursing and Midwifery Research Conference. Dublin; 2009

[220] McNulty CA, Bowen J, Foy C, Gunn K, Freeman E, Tompkins D, et al. Urinary catheterization in care homes for older people: Self-reported questionnaire audit of catheter management by care home staff. The Journal of Hospital Infection. 2006; **62**(1):29-36

[221] Fleming AA, Day J, Glanfield G. Registered nurse management of urinary catheters in a rehabilitation and long stay care hospital. International Journal of Nursing Practice. 2000;**6**(5):237-346

[222] Aldridge MD. Writing and designing readable patient education materials. Nephrology Nursing Journal. 2004;**31**(4):373-377

[223] Roy A, Abubakar I, Yates S, Chapman A, Lipman M, Monk P, et al. Evaluating knowledge gain from TB leaflets for prison and homeless sector staff: The National Knowledge Service TB pilot. European Journal of Public Health. 2008 Dec;**18**(6):600-603

[224] Saint S, Kowalski CP, Kaufman SR, Saint S, Kowalski CP, Kaufman SR, et al. Preventing hospital-acquired urinary tract infection in the United States: A national study. Clinical Infectious Diseases. 2008;**46**:243-250

[225] Nicolle LE, Bradley S, Colgan R, Nicolle LE, Bradley S, Colgan R, et al. Infectious Diseases Society of America guidelines for the diagnosis and treatment of asymptomatic bacteriuria in adults. Clinical Infectious Diseases. 2005;**40**:643-654

[226] Raz R, Schiller D, Nicolle LE. Chronic indwelling catheter replacement before antimicrobial therapy for

symptomatic urinary tract infection. The Journal of Urology. 2000;**164**:1254-1258

[227] Rodríguez-Baño J, Navarro MD, Retamar P, Picón E, Pascual A, the Extended-Spectrum Beta-Lactamases–Red Española de Investigación en Patología Infecciosa/Grupo de Estudio de Infeción Hospitalaria. Beta-lactam/Beta-lactam inhibitor combinations for the treatment of Bacteremia due to extended-Spectrum Beta-lactamase–producing Escherichia coli: A post hoc analysis of prospective cohorts. Clinical Infectious Diseases. 2012;**54**:167-174

[228] Tumbarello M, Trecarichi EM, De Rosa FG, Giannella M, Giacobbe DR, Bassetti M, et al. Infections caused by KPC-producing Klebsiella pneumoniae: Differences in therapy and mortality in a multicentre study. The Journal of Antimicrobial Chemotherapy. 2015;**70**(7):2133-2143

Chapter 3

Non-Microbiological Tests for the Diagnosis of Urinary Tract Infection

Laura Cristina Nocua-Báez and Jorge Alberto Cortés

Abstract

After clinical evaluation, suspicion of urinary tract infection might be modified by different tests that have the ability to augment (or diminish) the probability of a positive urinary culture and a confirmed diagnosis. In this review, we evaluate the possible role of different non microbiological test for the diagnosis of an urinary tract infection. Some of them might be easily available in the office or a busy emergency room, while others require more sophisticated infrastructure. Due to the high frequency of urinary tract infections, the diversity of symptoms, the difficulty of the diagnosis in some group of patients (e.g., older patients, those with dementia, etc.), and the lack of a gold standard, those non-microbiological tests might contribute to a correct diagnosis and a proper use of antibiotics in difficult cases.

Keywords: urinary tract infections, urine dipstick, biomarkers, renal gammagraphy, dipstick test

1. Introduction

Urinary tract infection (UTI) is an inflammation of the uroepithelial tissue, renal parenchyma or prostate resulting from pathological interaction with a microorganism. According to the anatomical location of the involvement, it might be divided into upper infection when it corresponds to pyelonephritis and lower, related to the renal pelvis or lower urinary tract, and refers almost exclusively to cystitis. Although this infectious disease is one of the most frequent reasons for consultation in all age groups, the most affected are women of reproductive age, with a peak between 14 and 24 years of age, due to the fact that sexual activity increases the probability of urovaginal colonization by Enterobacteriaceae present in the gastrointestinal tract. It is estimated that during their lifetime more than 60% of women may have at least one episode of urinary tract infection, and that it may recur 27% in the first 6 months, and more than once in 2.7% of patients [1].

The Enterobacterales group is the most frequent etiology of urinary tract infection, whose main pathogen is *Echerichia coli* in up to 90% of cases, followed by *Klebsiella spp, Proteus spp, Enterobacter spp, and Citrobacter spp*. Other microorganisms are *Enterococcus spp, Pseudomonas spp*, and *Staphylococcus saprophyticus*. UTI might be divided into complicated or uncomplicated, according to the presence of predisposing factors for failure of antimicrobial treatment such as anatomical or functional alterations of the urinary tract, pregnancy, and comorbidities such as diabetes mellitus [2]. The specific frequency of microorganisms for each group varies according to the clinical scenario, since in uncomplicated UTI, *E. coli* accounts for more than 90% of isolations, while in complicated UTI it is usually found in only 50 to 60% of patients.

In the diagnosis of UTI, the analysis of symptoms is fundamental; patients may present a variety of clinical manifestations, the finding of which is not specific. In general, it is important to consider differential diagnoses at the abdominal level, urological pathologies such as urolithiasis, genital pathology in women, and sexually transmitted diseases. The clinical presentation of the disease varies depending on the location; in the case of cystitis, the most important manifestations are the irritative symptoms of dysuria, tenesmus, hematuria, tenesmus, polyuria, and pollakiuria, in the absence of vaginal symptoms such as irritation or leucorrhea. Upper tract infection is characterized by systemic inflammatory signs such as fever (temperature greater than 38.3°C), tachycardia, tachypnea, nausea, and chills, which are accompanied by laboratory alterations such as leukocytosis or leukopenia; severe lumbar or abdominal pain may also occur. Approximately 30% of cases of high UTI are accompanied by irritative urinary symptoms [3]. Because of the broad clinical presentation and the nonspecificity of symptoms, the most important criterion for the diagnosis of UTI is the identification of bacteriuria, usually with elevated colony-forming unit counts (greater than 100, 1000 or 100,000 depending on the clinical scenario). However, although urine culture is fundamental for establishing the picture, the differential diagnosis is broad, and the frequency of bacteriuria without symptoms of cystitis is relatively frequent in patients with complicated infection. Therefore, to improve diagnostic certainty in the presence of bacteriuria and to support the rational use of antimicrobials, non-microbiological laboratory tools can be used to support the diagnosis. The aim of this chapter is precisely to describe the usefulness of several non-microbiological diagnostic tests that can help support the diagnosis of a urinary tract infection.

2. Limitations of bacteriuria identification

Given the need to establish bacteriuria as a fundamental element in the diagnosis of UTI, it is important to understand the limitations of its identification. Often, the presence of bacteriuria alone, in relation to unclear clinical pictures or patients at risk of poor progression (e.g., patients with Alzheimer's disease) is used as an argument for the use of antibiotics. This brings problems such as diagnostic uncertainty, poor clinical results, risk of bacterial resistance, and adverse effects derived from their use. This is the reason why additional tests may be required, hopefully with rapid results, to clearly differentiate the sick patient from the colonized one. Here, we will briefly describe the problems of sample collection and bacteriuria.

2.1 Collection and processing of the urine sample

The proper collection of a urine sample is of vital importance in the study of a UTI, and the spontaneous midstream urine collection technique is preferable. Another strategy is the use of an urinary catheter. However, this may increase the risk of development an infectious process, and it has been found that the use of catheter for the collection of the sample, even used only once, may favor the development of an infection in up to 1% of cases [4]. It is preferable to obtain the sample from the middle of the urinary stream in order to clean the urethra, which may be colonized by microorganisms not responsible for the clinical manifestations, at the beginning of urination. This strategy also favors the reduction of sample contamination that may be suspected with the finding of low epithelial cells and mucus in the urinary sediment. Some cleaning methods prior to sample collection have been used, such as washing the skin or periurethral mucous membranes, without finding consistent benefits for recommending it routinely [5]. In some cases, spontaneous sampling is difficult, especially in elderly patients or those with comorbidities involving compromised mobility, in which case the alternative is the use of catheterization. Suprapubic puncture is the method that best guarantees the absence of contamination of the sample, but it is uncomfortable, invasive, and impractical, so it is only used in very specific scenarios.

All samples should be processed as soon as possible and refrigerated, as bacteria can grow rapidly and their presence would be overestimated. Increases in the number of colony forming units (CFU) per ml greater than 10^5 CFU/mL have been documented 2–4 hours after collection, which increases the likelihood of false positives. The recommendation is to process the sample within 2 hours, otherwise refrigerate it or place it in a preservative. The processing of the sample for cultures corresponds to a microbiological test that is beyond the scope of this chapter. In general, it is considered the use of conventional media, semiquantitative methods, and an overnight incubation at 35–37°C in ambient air for a maximum of 48 hours or more in case of suspicion of fungal etiology [6, 7].

2.2 Bacteriuria, risk factors, and frequency

Traditionally it has been mentioned that urine is sterile in healthy individuals, without comorbidity. However, studies have identified bacteriuria in up to 5% of non-pregnant premenopausal women [8], and a complete microbiota related to urine has been recently identified [9]. Other classical risk factors for bacteriuria include urinary tract catheterization. Short-term use of bladder catheters may be associated with bacteriuria in relation to device care and duration of use. It is estimated that between 9 and 23% of patients may acquire bacteriuria as a result of device use [10]. Most patients resolve bacteriuria after device removal; however, a proportion may end up with a urinary tract infection that becomes clinically evident within 48 hours. Predictors of bacteriuria include ICU stay and a duration of the device for more than 10 days [11]. In fact, catheters of long duration, greater than 30 days, are considered to have a colonization frequency close to 100%, independent of other care measures. Intermittent catheterization in individuals who have spinal cord injury and require it for problems related to neurogenic bladder may have a frequency of bacteriuria ranging from 23 to 69%. Age, comorbidity, and site of care also have an effect on the frequency of bacteriuria: Postmenopausal women increase the frequency of bacteriuria in relation to decades of life and can reach 20% in those over 80 years of age. However, in the latter scenario, it is confounded by comorbidity and site of care [10]. Patients with diabetes may have a prevalence of bacteriuria that can reach 27%, while men or women residing in nursing homes or chronic care settings may have a frequency of up to 40 or 60%, respectively [10].

3. Non-microbiologic urine tests for the diagnosis of urinary tract infection

3.1 Urinalysis

Macroscopic and microscopic analysis of urine includes several parameters. Relevant information on each of them is presented below:

3.1.1 Color, odor, and pH

There are several initial characteristics to evaluate in a urine sample, such as color, odor, and pH. A change in odor does not suggest infection; finding it "strong" is usually due to a concentrated sample, although the presence of UTI may give a pungent odor. There are findings in urine color that may be nonspecifically related to infection, such as cloudy for pyuria, greenish or blue for *Pseudomonas spp,* purple for *Proteus spp, Morganella spp, Providencia spp*, and even *E. coli* (product of tryptophan metabolism to indoxyl sulfate) and red in relation to hematuria [12–14]. Normal urinary pH is slightly acidic between 4.5 and 5.5; alkalinization of urine may occur in the case of urolithiasis due to magnesium and ammonium phosphate crystals, due to infection related to microorganisms that interfere with urea metabolism, such as *Proteus spp* [12].

3.1.2 Pyuria by direct microscopy

Pyuria supports the diagnosis of urinary tract inflammation, although it is not a specific element of infection because other pathologies can cause it, such as non-infectious prostatitis, urolithiasis, postoperative abdominal or pelvic procedures, use of urinary devices, sexually transmitted diseases, trauma, or sepsis. The absence of pyuria in patients decreases the likelihood of an infectious process in light of the relevant clinical elements; but it cannot be considered alone for the analysis of absence of disease. For the search of pyuria in the microscopic study of urine, the sample must be rapidly processed, in less than two hours, because of the accelerated deterioration of leukocytes. It is possible to directly observe leukocytes and leukocyte casts that can be counted in a centrifuged sample or with Gram stain. In general, counts greater than 2 leukocytes/mm^3 are suggestive of inflammation, which, as noted, does not necessarily refer to infection. The most accurate test for the detection of pyuria is the measurement of the urinary leukocyte excretion rate, with a cut-off point for infection greater than 400. 000 leukocytes/hour, but this is not routinely used because of the impracticality of its realization; for this reason, it has been opted for the counting of cells with hemocytometers, where the correlation with the cut-off point of the leukocyte excretion rate and with significant Gram bacteriuria $\geq 10^5$CFU/ml is $\geqslant 10$ leukocytes/mm3; counts of 8–10 cells/mm3 have been correlated with values below $<10^5$CFU/ml in samples without contamination by suprapubic aspiration in patients with dysuria [15, 16].

3.1.3 Bacteriuria (without culture): direct microscopy and gram staining

The finding of bacteria in the examination of a urine specimen is the main aid in the diagnosis of UTI. Bacteria can be observed directly in the sediment of an uncentrifuged specimen or with Gram staining, the later being the most relevant method. Gram staining is simple and allows an early approach to the diagnosis of infection; it can even guide empirical antimicrobial treatment based on the characterization of infectious agents as Gram-positive or Gram-negative. The cut-off values of CFU/ml are not entirely standardized, and the main studies on their diagnostic performance are old. Significant bacteriuria without symptoms is defined as a repeated finding in women of $\geq 10^5$ CFU/ml in a midstream urine specimen; in pregnant women, of more than $\geq 10^3$ CFU/ml; and in men, of a specimen with $\geq 10^5$ CFU/ml. For patients with symptoms, bacteriuria is significant with a finding on midstream urine collection in women $\geq 10^3$ CFU/ml and in men $\geq 10^2$ CFU/ml. For these cut-off points, different diagnostic yields have been reported with a sensitivity between 81 and 97% and specificity between 71 and 96%, [17–21].

3.2 Dipstick test

The dipstick allows the detection of enzyme activity in patients with suspected UTI such as nitrites from bacterial nitrate reductase activity, leukocyte elastase from leukocytes that are presumably active in the infected urinary tract, and the presence of red blood cells in relation to hematuria due to inflammation of the urinary tract. The dipstick has become a noninvasive, practical, and rapid tool that supports the diagnosis of an infection and can guide early decisions to initiate empirical antimicrobial treatment, but should always be interpreted in conjunction with the clinical picture of the patients.

3.2.1 Nitrite test

Urinary tract infection is often associated with the presence of nitrite in the urine as a result of bacterial nitrate reductase enzyme activity on nitrates [22]. The uropathogens that most cause UTI are nitrite producers; however, other microorganisms such as *Enterococcus spp, Pseudomonas spp, Streptococcus saprophyticus*, and other non-fermenting microorganisms do not produce it. One of the difficulties of this test is that it should ideally be performed after at least 4 hours without urination, because it requires the time necessary for the production of nitrites in the bladder by bacteria. The diagnostic performance of the nitrite test in correlation with significant bacteriuria in patients with UTI has been analyzed in several studies with variable findings, reaching sensitivity values of 70.5% and specificity of 58% [23]. However, sensitivity might be as low as 28.9% [24]. In a meta-analysis that included various population groups such as the elderly, children, pregnant women and the general population, a sensitivity of 40 to 60%, and a specificity of 85 to 98% were found, with the best performance in the elderly and the worst in pregnant women [25]. Therefore, its most important value is its positive predictive value.

3.2.2 Leukocyte esterase test

The leukocyte esterase test suggests pyuria in urine, its basis is the hydrolysis of ester substrates by the stereolytic activity of enzymes present in leukocytes that produce alcohols and acids, mainly in neutrophils, which have more than 10 proteins with this function. The positive result is evidenced by a change in the color of the test strip whose intensity is proportional to the amount of pyuria, due to the presence of resting or active leukocytes. The main false-positives of the test are the presence of bacteria in the vaginal discharge, parasites such as Trichomonas and eosinophils.

The most frequent false-negatives are high levels of protein or glucose, use of boric acid preservatives or large amounts of ascorbic or oxalic acid [6]. The diagnostic yield of leukocyte esterase is good in patients with suspected UTI in correlation with bacteriuria, with sensitivity varying from 72% to 97.5% and specificity from 74.5% to 84.7% [26, 27]. In association with UTI, a sensitivity of 64% and specificity of 73% has been documented. This performance varies according to the sampling setting; in primary care the sensitivity is 76%, while in tertiary care units it is 62%. Due to the fact that the reading of the test is observer dependent, if the physician is the one who performs it, the sensitivity is 86%; in the case of the test performed by nursing group, the sensitivity lowers to 67%, while if it is done by laboratory personnel, the resulting sensitivity is 59%. Therefore, the professional involved in the interpretation of the test strip must be well trained [28].

3.2.3 Leukocyte esterase and nitrites

The positive result of leukocyte esterase and nitrite simultaneously could further support the diagnosis; this has been evaluated in several studies where it has been found that the combination of these positive tests increases the sensitivity from 68–88%, with a variable performance in specificity. These findings appear to be more accurate in urology patients. However, it is not clear that finding these two positive tests together helps to clarify the diagnosis of UTI or asymptomatic bacteriuria [28–30]. The finding of a negative result of both tests helps to rule out infection, due to their high negative predictive value; however, the interpretation must be made taking into account the clinical scenario and the suspicion of differential diagnoses [25].

4. Acute phase reactants serum tests

4.1 C-reactive protein

C-reactive protein (CRP) is a pentraxin that is released by the liver as part of the acute response to damage such as infection or inflammation, which has proven useful in the diagnosis of different infectious processes; in UTI it can support the anatomical location of the infection, the highest values have been correlated with acute pyelonephritis. Levels of 113.48 mg/L are associated with upper UTI versus 12.84 ± mg/L for those with lower tract infection. CRP has also been reported to be between 126.6 and 127.33 mg/L for upper UTI and between 4.7 and 14.5 mg/L for lower UTI. Attempts have been made to establish cut-off points for this biomarker in relation to upper UTI, finding that levels above 100 mg/L may be useful for this diagnosis [31, 32]. The performance of CRP with a cut-off point of 20 mg/L for acute pyelonephritis in adults has a sensitivity of 85.71% and specificity of 48%. However, in the search for the degree of renal damage related to the differentiation between tissue invasion by the microorganism vs. only cystitis, there is no clear usefulness of the role of this biomarker [33]. In children, a Cochrane meta-analysis found that a CRP value of 20 mg/L had a sensitivity of 94% and specificity of 39% for the diagnosis of acute pyelonephritis [34].

4.2 Procalcitonin

Procalcitonin (PCT) is a calcitonin precursor protein free of hormonal activity, used for the early diagnosis of bacterial infections and sepsis; it is also useful for the correlation with the severity of disease and therefore corresponds to a prognostic predictor [35]. PCT is generally elevated in systemic involvement and not in localized infection such as cystitis. This biomarker is increased in acute pyelonephritis with a variable sensitivity and specificity ranging between 70 and 100% and between 70 and 95%, respectively [36, 37]. In a study performed with children where PCT was compared for the early diagnosis of UTI with CRP, erythrocyte sedimentation rate (ESR) and leukocyte count, with a cut-off value greater than 0.85 μg/L, it had a better performance with a sensitivity of 89%, a specificity of 97% and positive and negative predictive values of 96% and 91%, respectively [38]. Another benefit of the use of PCT in adults in this context is the prediction of secondary bacteremia that occurs in up to 23% of patients; a level higher than 0,25 μg/L has a sensitivity of 95% and a specificity of 50% for this clinical presentation, so PCT values could be helpful for early identification of complications of acute pyelonephritis that lead to longer hospital stay, mortality, and health care costs. A PCT level ≤ 0,25 μg/L reduces the use of blood cultures by up to 40%, with a loss in the detection of bacteremia of 3% [39]. It is worth remembering that PCT elevates its value in patients with renal failure (acute or chronic) and is not interpretable in patients with creatinine levels above 1.5 mg/dl. Currently, the available information on PCT in adults with pyelonephritis could not be used to generate a clear recommendation.

4.3 Other biomarkers in urinary tract infection

Due to the low specificity and intermediate sensitivity of non-microbiological tests for the diagnosis of UTI such as leukocyte esterase, nitrites, pyuria, PCT, and CRP, which even lead to overtreatment in up to 43% of patients and undertreatment in 13% [40], with consequences such as high recurrence, prolonged hospital stays, increased bacterial resistance and renal damage, in recent years there has been increased interest in the search for diagnostic tests that are reliable and easily performed.

One of the biomarkers is neutrophil gelatinase-associated lipocalin (NGAL), which is also an acute phase protein like CRP; it rises after 12 hours from the onset of a UTI, and its maximum peak occurs at 72 hours; it can be measured in serum or urine, and in the later, it is even a predictor of the resolution of the infection and at the same time of its duration [41]. One of the advantages of the use of NGAL is that it is not influenced by the glomerular filtration rate unlike CRP and PCT, but apparently it does not allow to establish the localization of the infectious process [42].

Another group of promising biomarkers are the cytokines present in all infectious and inflammatory processes, which could have a good sensitivity for UTI with an intermediate specificity. The most studied are interleukin 1-beta (IL-1ß) in urine and serum, and in children a value in urine greater than 150 pg./mL for the diagnosis of acute pyelonephritis has a sensitivity of 79% and a specificity of 88% [43]. Interleukin 6 (IL-6) in urine in elderly adult patients with a cut-off level of 30 pg./mL allows differentiation of acute pyelonephritis from asymptomatic bacteriuria with a sensitivity of 80% and a specificity of 82%, while its usefulness in defining UTI vs. asymptomatic bacteriuria has a sensitivity of 48% [44, 45]. Regarding interleukin-8 (IL-8) in urine, a value higher than 200 pg./mL in children indicates a UTI, with a sensitivity of 93% and a specificity of 90% [46].

Other tests have been studied such as heparin-binding protein product of neutrophil activation, matrix metalloprotease-9 (MMP-9) whose increase occurs simultaneously with NGAL, lactoferrin, and heat shock protein-70 which appear to be promising [47].

5. Imaging tests

Although diagnostic imaging has traditionally been considered in the context of suspected complicated pyelonephritis as a strategy for the identification of comorbidities that may explain the presence of the infection, in some complex scenarios its use may be considered to reach the diagnosis.

5.1 Renal ultrasound

Some authors recommend early imaging as a strategy for the timely detection of complications or confirmation of the suspicion of acute pyelonephritis, but it is considered that new and significant abnormal findings will be found in only 16% of patients; therefore, it is necessary to perform new studies that evaluate cost–benefit [48]. One of the most readily available imaging tests is ultrasonography (US), which allows an initial approach, with findings such as hydronephrosis, obstructive uropathy, papillary necrosis, renal abscess, local nephritis, inflammation of the perirenal fat, and emphysematous pyelonephritis. One study found a sensitivity of ultrasonography of only 33% compared to tomography for the diagnosis of acute pyelonephritis [49]. Now the use of contrast has been added to US, finding that compared to scintigraphy marked with dimercaptosuccinic acid and technetium 99 m (Tc-DMSA and 99mTc), the sensitivity of this test is 86.8%, and the specificity is 71.4% [50].

5.2 Computerized axial tomography

Another imaging technique for the diagnosis of high UTI is computed tomography (CT). The most frequently described findings for the diagnostic support of the infectious disease are the presence of localized hypodense lesions, product of renal ischemia due to infiltration of immune system cells such as neutrophils and lymphocytes, parenchymal edema, and perirenal fat and/or gas (suggestive of emphysematous pyelonephritis or abscesses). In a study with 24 patients with acute pyelonephritis, a correlation between CT and scintigraphy marked with DMSA and 99mTc was found in 11 cases, but 11 of the remaining 13 had an abnormal CT with normal scintigraphy, concluding that tomography has greater precision compared to scintigraphy [51]. CT vs. US has a sensitivity of 81% vs. 33% for the diagnosis of acute pyelonephritis [49]. In children the diagnosis of this infection is even more difficult, so imaging strategies have greater importance, one of the most used is the DMSA scan, which has been compared with CT, finding that the latter has the advantage of differentiating and determining the local inflammatory changes of the renal parenchyma that in the scan may go unnoticed [52].

5.3 Nuclear magnetic resonance imaging (NMR)

Magnetic resonance imaging is an imaging test that has the advantage of not using radiation, but may not be readily available in all clinical settings. Alterations in patients with acute pyelonephritis include areas of hyperintensity or hypointensity, decrease or loss of normal corticomedullary differentiation, scarring, complications such as perirenal fluid, collections or abscesses and gas. This diagnostic tool can also differentiate acute lesions from scarring, which cannot be determined with conventional nuclear medicine techniques. The diagnostic performance of this test in patients with acute pyelonephritis has shown a sensitivity of 96% and a specificity of

86% [53]. Another study showed a sensitivity of 89,5% and specificity of 87,5% for NMR and a S of 86,8% and E of 87,5% for computed tomography [49].

5.4 Nuclear medicine: radioactive isotope scintigraphy

Scintigraphy labeled with radioactive isotopes such as DMSA and 99mTc is a test that has been used mainly in pediatric patients in order to identify renal involvement and to define prognosis. Its use in adults has been limited. This diagnostic tool is useful to determine the functional renal tubular mass, so its great advantage is to detect regional damage, specially cortical involvement. There is consensus on its use in the search for renal scarring, for example, after acute pyelonephritis, but its diagnostic capacity for acute events is controversial. Single photon emission computed tomography (SPECT) is another scintigraphy technique, which is also more popular in the pediatric setting. In animal models when comparing SPECT vs. CT vs. MRI for the diagnosis of acute pyelonephritis, SPECT has a sensitivity of 92.1% and a specificity of 93.8%, MR of 89,5% and 87,5%, CT of 88,2% and 93,5%, and US of 56,6% and 81,4%, respectively [54]. For the detection of acute pyelonephritis, in the comparison of the use of planar or standard DMSA vs. SPECT, the latter technique has a sensitivity of 97% and specificity of 66%, vs. 82% and 97%, respectively, for standard DMSA [55].

In **Table 1**, the diagnostic performance of the different non-microbiological tests for urinary tract infection is summarized. Cut-off points and specific test findings are given in the text.

Diagnostic test	Sensibility% (Range%)	Specificity% (Range %)	Clinical scenario	Reference
Pyuria (⩾10 leukocytes/mm3)	85 (75–96)	96 (94–98)	Patients with significant bacteriuria ≥105 CFU/ml as diagnostic criteria for UTI.	[16]
Bacteriuria in urine Gram (⩾105 CFU/mL)	89 (81–97)	93 (91–96)	Adults with a clinical diagnosis of UTI and a positive urine culture	[10, 17, 18, 20, 21]
Dipstick: nitrites	50 (40–60)	91 (85–98)	Children, adults, elderly, and pregnant women with UTI	[28]
Dipstick: esterase	85 (72–97,5)	84 (74,5-84,7)	Adults and elderly with significant bacteriuria ≥105 CFU/ml and symptoms of UTI	[27, 28]
Dipstick: nitrites and esterase	78 (68–88)	62 (55–87)	Adults with significant bacteriuria ≥105 CFU/ml and symptoms of UTI.	[28, 30]
C-reactive protein ⩾ 20 mg/L	94 (85–97)	39 (23–58)	Children	[34]
C-reactive protein ⩾ 6.5 mg/L	57,2 (48.9–65.4)	54,4 (51.8–57.0)	Adults aged ≥65 years	[56]
Procalcitonin ⩾ 0.5 μg/L	86 (72–93)	74 (55–87)	Children	[34]
Procalcitonin ⩾ 0.25 μg/L	95 (89–98)	50 (46–55)	Adults with bacteremia secondary to UTI	[39]

Diagnostic test	Sensibility% (Range%)	Specificity% (Range %)	Clinical scenario	Reference
Interleukin 1-beta (IL-1B) ⩾ 150 pg./ml	79	88	Children with acute pyelonephritis	[43]
Interleukin 6 (IL-6) ⩾ 30 pg./ml	80	86	Elderly with acute pyelonephritis	[44]
Interleukin 8 (IL-8) ⩾ 200 pg./ml	93	90	Children	[46]
Ultrasonography with contrast	86,8	71,4	Children with acute pyelonephritis vs. Tc-DMSA and 99mTc	[50]
Computerized axial tomography	81	—	Adults with acute pyelonephritis vs. US and vs. DMSA	[49]
Nuclear magnetic resonance	96	86	Adults with acute pyelonephritis vs. CT scan	[53]

Table 1.
Diagnostic yield of non-microbiological tests for urinary tract infection.

6. Conclusions

Urinary tract infection is a common disease in all age ranges, which requires early diagnosis for timely treatment to reduce patient complications. There are several non-microbiological tests available that support the diagnosis of this infection and decision making for the start of empirical antimicrobial treatment; the most commonly used are direct microscopy of the urine sample, Gram stain and dipstick, all of which should always be interpreted with the clinical manifestations of the patients. The most important finding is the presence of bacteria in the urine sample. There are several biomarkers that can aid in UTI diagnosis, localization and prognosis of patients, such as CRP; promising new biomarkers that may contribute to diagnosis are being studied, such as NGAL, IL-1ß, IL-6, and IL-8. Imaging techniques are also tools for the diagnosis of UTI, with greater importance in the search for complications or associated structural or functional alterations, and limited information for their routine use in clinical settings.

Author details

Laura Cristina Nocua-Báez[1] and Jorge Alberto Cortés[1,2]*

1 Facultad de Medicina, Department of Internal Medicine, Universidad Nacional de Colombia, Sede Bogotá, Bogotá, Colombia

2 Infectious Diseases Unit, Hospital Universitario Nacional, Bogotá, Colombia

*Address all correspondence to: jacortesl@unal.edu.co

References

[1] Medina M, Castillo-Pino E. An introduction to the epidemiology and burden of urinary tract infections. Therapeutic Advances in Urology. 2019;**11**:1756287219832172. DOI: 10.1177/1756287219832172

[2] Klein RD, Hultgren SJ. Urinary tract infections: Microbial pathogenesis, host pathogen interactions and new treatment strategies. Nature Reviews. Microbiology. 2020;**18**(4):211-226. DOI: 10.1038/s41579-020-0324-0

[3] Johnson JR, Russo TA. Acute pyelonephritis in adults. The New England Journal of Medicine. 2018;**378**(1):48-59. DOI: 10.1056/nejmcp1702758

[4] Cuervo Maldonado Sonia Isabel, Alberto Cortés Luna Jorge Alberto. Nosocomial Urinary Tract Infections [Internet]. 2010. Available from: www.intechopen.com

[5] Lifshitz E, Kramer L. Outpatient urine culture: does collection technique matter? Archives of Internal Medicine. 2000;**160**(16):2537-2540. DOI: 10.1001/archinte.160.16.2537

[6] Wilson ML, Gaido L. Laboratory diagnosis of urinary tract infections in adult patients. Clinical Infectious Diseases. 2004;**38**(8):1150-1158. DOI: 10.1086/383029

[7] Silver SA, Baillie L, Simor AE. Positive urine cultures: A major cause of inappropriate antimicrobial use in hospitals? Canadian Journal of Infectious Diseases and Medical Microbiology. 2009;**20**(4):107-111. DOI: 10.1155/2009/702545

[8] Hooton TM, Roberts PL, Stapleton AE. Asymptomatic bacteriuria and pyuria in premenopausal women. Clinical Infectious Diseases. 2021;**72**(8):1332-1338. DOI: 10.1093/cid/ciaa274

[9] Perez-Carrasco V, Soriano-Lerma A, Soriano M, Gutiérrez-Fernández J, Garcia-Salcedo JA. Urinary microbiome: Yin and Yang of the urinary tract. Frontiers in Cellular and Infection Microbiology. 2021;**18**(11):617002. DOI: 10.3389/fcimb.2021.617002

[10] Colgan R, Nicolle LE, Mcglone A, Hooton TM. Asymptomatic Bacteriuria in Adults. American Family Physician. 2006;**74**(6):985-990

[11] Ortiz-Ramirez L et al. Factores asociados: características clínicas, microbiológicas y perfiles de resistencia en infecciones urinarias asociadas a catéter en dos hospitales de alta complejidad. Infection. 2022;**26**(2):161-167. DOI: 10.22354/inv26i2.1016

[12] Simerville JA, Maxted WC, Pahira JJ. Urinalysis: A comprehensive review. American Family Physician. 2005;**71**(6):1153-1162

[13] Raymond JR, Yarger WE. Abnormal urine color: differential diagnosis. Southern Medical Journal. 1988;**81**(7):837-841. DOI: 10.1097/00007611-198807000-00008

[14] Aycock RD, Kass DA. Abnormal urine color. Southern Medical Journal. 2012;**105**(1):43-47. DOI: 10.1097/SMJ.0b013e31823c413e

[15] Stamm WE, Counts GW, Running KR, Fihn S, Turck M, Holmes KK. Diagnosis of coliform infection in acutely dysuric women. The New England Journal of Medicine.

1982;**307**(8):463-468. DOI: 10.1056/NEJM198208193070802

[16] Pappas PG. Laboratory in the diagnosis and management of urinary tract infections. The Medical Clinics of North America. 1991;**75**(2):313-325. DOI: 10.1016/s0025-7125(16)30456-4

[17] Tilton RE, Tilton RC. Automated direct antimicrobial susceptibility testing of microscopically screened urine cultures. Journal of Clinical Microbiology. 1980;**11**(2):157-161. DOI: 10.1128/jcm.11.2.157-161.1980

[18] Winquist AG, Orrico MA, Peterson LR. Evaluation of the cytocentrifuge gram stain as a screening test for bacteriuria in specimens from specific patient populations. American Journal of Clinical Pathology. 1997;**108**(5):515-524. DOI: 10.1093/ajcp/108.5.515

[19] Nicolle LE, Bradley S, Colgan R, Rice JC, Schaeffer A, Hooton TM. Infectious Diseases Society of America; American Society of Nephrology; American geriatric society. Infectious Diseases Society of America guidelines for the diagnosis and treatment of asymptomatic bacteriuria in adults. Clinical Infectious Diseases. 2005;**40**(5):643-654. DOI: 10.1086/427507

[20] Cardoso CL, Muraro CB, Siqueira VL, Guilhermetti M. Simplified technique for detection of significant bacteriuria by microscopic examination of urine. Journal of Clinical Microbiology. 1998;**36**(3):820-823. DOI: 10.1128/JCM.36.3.820-823.1998

[21] McNair RD, MacDonald SR, Dooley SL, Peterson LR. Evaluation of the centrifuged and gram-stained smear, urinalysis, and reagent strip testing to detect asymptomatic bacteriuria in obstetric patients. American Journal of Obstetrics and Gynecology. 2000;**182**(5):1076-1079. DOI: 10.1067/mob.2000.105440

[22] Lundberg JO, Carlsson S, Engstrand L, Morcos E, Wiklund NP, Weitzberg E. Urinary nitrite: More than a marker of infection. Urology. 1997;**50**(2):189-191. DOI: 10.1016/S0090-4295(97)00257-4

[23] Bafna P, Deepanjali S, Mandal J, Balamurugan N, Swaminathan RP, Kadhiravan T. Reevaluating the true diagnostic accuracy of dipstick tests to diagnose urinary tract infection using Bayesian latent class analysis. PLoS One. 2020;**15**(12):e0244870. DOI: 10.1371/journal.pone.0244870

[24] Coulthard MG. Using urine nitrite sticks to test for urinary tract infection in children aged < 2 years: A meta-analysis. Pediatric Nephrology. 2019;**34**(7):1283-1288. DOI: 10.1007/s00467-019-04226-6

[25] Bellazreg F, Abid M, Lasfar NB, Hattab Z, Hachfi W, Letaief A. Diagnostic value of dipstick test in adult symptomatic urinary tract infections: Results of a cross-sectional Tunisian study. The Pan African Medical Journal. 2019;**21**(33):131. DOI: 10.11604/pamj.2019.33.131.17190

[26] Nava MO, Mirzaei N, Ebrahimian V, Molaei M, Tohidnia F, Pursafar M. Diagnostic value of leukocyte esterase and nitrite tests for the detection of urinary tract infection. Biomedical and Pharmacology Journal. 2012;**5**(2):1-4

[27] Oneson R, Gröschel DH. Leukocyte esterase activity and nitrite test as a rapid screen for significant bacteriuria. American Journal of Clinical Pathology. 1985;**83**(1):84-87. DOI: 10.1093/ajcp/83.1.84

[28] Devillé WL, Yzermans JC, van Duijn NP, Bezemer PD, van der Windt DA, Bouter LM. The urine dipstick test useful to rule out infections. A meta-analysis of the accuracy. BMC Urology. 2004;**4**:4. DOI: 10.1186/1471-2490-4-4

[29] Semeniuk H, Church D. Evaluation of the leukocyte esterase and nitrite urine dipstick screening tests for detection of bacteriuria in women with suspected uncomplicated urinary tract infections. Journal of Clinical Microbiology. 1999;**37**(9):3051-3052. DOI: 10.1128/JCM.37.9.3051-3052.1999

[30] Mambatta AK, Jayarajan J, Rashme VL, Harini S, Menon S, Kuppusamy J. Reliability of dipstick assay in predicting urinary tract infection. Journalof Family Medicine and Primary Care. 2015;**4**(2):265-268. DOI: 10.4103/2249-4863.154672

[31] Agrawal P, Pandey A, Sompura S, Pursnani ML. Role of blood C - reactive protein levels in upper urinary tract infection and lower urinary tract infection in adult patients (>16 years). The Journal of the Association of Physicians of India. 2013;**61**(7): 462-463

[32] Narayan Swamy SN, Jakanur RK, Sangeetha SR. Significance of C-reactive protein levels in categorizing upper and lower urinary tract infection in adult patients. Cureus. 2022;**14**(6):e26432. DOI: 10.7759/cureus.26432

[33] Xu RY, Liu HW, Liu JL, Dong JH. Procalcitonin and C-reactive protein in urinary tract infection diagnosis. BMC Urology. 2014;**14**:45. DOI: 10.1186/1471-2490-14-45

[34] Shaikh N, Borrell JL, Evron J, Leeflang MM. Procalcitonin, C-reactive protein, and erythrocyte sedimentation rate for the diagnosis of acute pyelonephritis in children. Cochrane Database of Systematic Reviews 2015;1(1):CD009185. DOI: 10.1002/14651858.CD009185.pub2

[35] Harbarth S, Holeckova K, Froidevaux C, Pittet D, Ricou B, Grau GE, et al. Diagnostic value of procalcitonin, interleukin-6, and interleukin-8 in critically ill patients admitted with suspected sepsis. American Journal of Respiratory and Critical Care Medicine. 2001;**164**(3):396-402. DOI: 10.1164/ajrccm.164.3.2009052

[36] Kotoula A, Gardikis S, Tsalkidis A, Mantadakis E, Zissimopoulos A, Kambouri K, et al. Procalcitonin for the early prediction of renal parenchymal involvement in children with UTI: Preliminary results. International Urology and Nephrology. 2009;**41**(2):393-399. DOI: 10.1007/s11255-008-9472-2

[37] Bharath MS et al. Role of procalcitonin and C-reactive protein in urinary tract infection diagnosis in adults. International Journal of Advances in Medicine. 2017;**4**(2):417-419. DOI: 10.18203/2349-3933.ijam20171001

[38] Kotoula A, Gardikis S, Tsalkidis A, Mantadakis E, Zissimopoulos A, Deftereos S, et al. Comparative efficacies of procalcitonin and conventional inflammatory markers for prediction of renal parenchymal inflammation in pediatric first urinary tract infection. Urology. 2009;**73**(4):782-786. DOI: 10.1016/j.urology.2008.10.042

[39] van Nieuwkoop C, Bonten TN, Van't Wout JW, Kuijper EJ, Groeneveld GH, Becker MJ, et al. Procalcitonin reflects bacteremia and bacterial load in urosepsis syndrome: A prospective observational study. Critical Care. 2010;**14**(6):R206. DOI: 10.1186/cc9328

[40] Hannula A, Perhomaa M, Venhola M, Pokka T, Renko M, Uhari M. Long-term follow-up of patients after childhood urinary tract infection. Archives of Pediatrics & Adolescent Medicine. 2012;**166**(12):1117-1122. DOI: 10.1001/archpediatrics.2012.1383

[41] Jung N, Byun HJ, Park JH, Kim JS, Kim HW, Ha JY. Diagnostic accuracy of urinary biomarkers in infants younger than 3 months with urinary tract infection. Korean Journal of Pediatrics. 2018;**61**(1):24-29. DOI: 10.3345/kjp.2018.61.1.24

[42] Urbschat A, Obermüller N, Paulus P, Reissig M, Hadji P, Hofmann R, et al. Upper and lower urinary tract infections can be detected early but not be discriminated by urinary NGAL in adults. International Urology and Nephrology. 2014;**46**(12):2243-2249. DOI: 10.1007/s11255-014-0831-x

[43] Sheu JN, Chen MC, Cheng SL, Lee IC, Chen SM, Tsay GJ. Urine interleukin-1beta in children with acute pyelonephritis and renal scarring. Nephrology (Carlton, Vic.). 2007;**12**(5):487-493. DOI: 10.1111/j.1440-1797.2007.00819.x

[44] Kjölvmark C, Tschernij E, Öberg J, Påhlman LI, Linder A, Åkesson P. Distinguishing asymptomatic bacteriuria from urinary tract infection in the elderly - the use of urine levels of heparin-binding protein and interleukin-6. Diagnostic Microbiology and Infectious Disease. 2016;**85**(2):243-248. DOI: 10.1016/j.diagmicrobio.2016.03.005

[45] Sundén F, Wullt B. Predictive value of urinary interleukin-6 for symptomatic urinary tract infections in a nursing home population. International Journal of Urology. 2016;**23**(2):168-174. DOI: 10.1111/iju.13002

[46] Rao WH, Evans GS, Finn A. The significance of interleukin 8 in urine. Archives of Disease in Childhood. 2001;**85**(3):256-262. DOI: 10.1136/adc.85.3.256

[47] Horváth J, Wullt B, Naber KG, Köves B. Biomarkers in urinary tract infections - which ones are suitable for diagnostics and follow-up? GMS Infectious Diseases. 2020;**26**(8):Doc24. DOI: 10.3205/id000068

[48] Shen Y, Brown MA. Renal imaging in pyelonephritis. Nephrology (Carlton, Vic.). 2004;**9**(1):22-25. DOI: 10.1111/j.1440-1797.2003.00226.x

[49] Yoo JM, Koh JS, Han CH, Lee SL, Ha US, Kang SH, et al. Diagnosing acute pyelonephritis with CT, Tc-DMSA SPECT, and Doppler ultrasound: A comparative study. Korean Journal of Urology. 2010;**51**(4):260-265. DOI: 10.4111/kju.2010.51.4.260

[50] Jung HJ, Choi MH, Pai KS, Kim HG. Diagnostic performance of contrast-enhanced ultrasound for acute pyelonephritis in children. Scientific Reports. 2020;**10**(1):10715. DOI: 10.1038/s41598-020-67713-z

[51] Sattari A, Kampouridis S, Damry N, Hainaux B, Ham HR, Vandewalle JC, et al. CT and 99mTc-DMSA scintigraphy in adult acute pyelonephritis: A comparative study. Journal of Computer Assisted Tomography. 2000;**24**(4):600-604. DOI: 10.1097/00004728-200007000-00016

[52] Lee J, Kwon DG, Park SJ, Pai KS. Discordant findings on dimercaptosuccinic acid scintigraphy in children with multi-detector row computed tomography-proven acute pyelonephritis. Korean Journal of Pediatrics. 2011;**54**(5):212-218. DOI: 10.3345/kjp.2011.54.5.212

[53] Sriman R, Venkatesh K, Mathew C, Pankaj M, Shankar R. Validity of diffusion-weighted magnetic resonance imaging in the evaluation of acute pyelonephritis in comparison with contrast-enhanced computed tomography. Polish Journal of Radiology. 2020;**85**:e137-e143. DOI: 10.5114/pjr.2020.93669

[54] Majd M, Nussbaum Blask AR, Markle BM, Shalaby-Rana E, Pohl HG, Park JS, et al. Acute pyelonephritis: Comparison of diagnosis with 99mTc-DMSA, SPECT, spiral CT, MR imaging, and power Doppler US in an experimental pig model. Radiology. 2001;**218**(1):101-108. DOI: 10.1148/radiology.218.1.r01ja37101

[55] Craig JC, Wheeler DM, Irwig L, Howman-Giles RB. How accurate is dimercaptosuccinic acid scintigraphy for the diagnosis of acute pyelonephritis? A meta-analysis of experimental studies. Journal of Nuclear Medicine. 2000;**41**(6):986-993

[56] Kuil SD, Hidad S, Fischer JC, Harting J, Hertogh CMPM, Prins JM, et al. Sensitivity of C-reactive protein and Procalcitonin measured by point-of-care tests to diagnose urinary tract infections in nursing home residents: A cross-sectional study. Clinical Infectious Diseases. 2021;**73**(11):e3867-e3875. DOI: 10.1093/cid/ciaa1709

Section 2

Challenges in Urinalysis

Chapter 4

Role of Urine Examination in Renal Transplant Recipients

Lovelesh K. Nigam

Abstract

Kidney transplantation has emerged as a major advance of modern medicine, providing high-quality life years to patients with end-stage renal disease (ESRD). Post-transplant monitoring of the transplanted kidney is based on physical examination, urine volume, the assessment of albuminuria or proteinuria, serum creatinine, and glomerular filtration rate (GFR) estimation based on serum creatinine. Of these multiple investigations, serum creatinine and urine analysis is one of the most widely used and accepted tool to assess graft dysfunction as well as plan management. Various immunological (rejections-antibody, cellular) and non-immunological (polyoma virus nephropathy, mycosis, recurrent/de novo diseases) may affect the graft function. Changes in various parameters like urine osmolality, proteinuria, hematuria and presence of casts, crystals and other cellular constituents aids in diagnosis diseases of the allograft. This chapter thus highlights the importance of most frequent parameters that help in assessing the graft function. In addition to these parameters, a brief introduction of biomarkers is also included. Many studies have shown that these biomarkers have a promising role in diagnosis of allograft disease and thus avoiding interventional procedures like renal biopsy. Easy availability as well as low-cost of the urine examination makes it a promising tool for overall assessment of the graft dysfunction.

Keywords: renal transplant, proteinuria, hematura, rejection, tubular injury, biomarkers

1. Introduction

Kidney transplantation has emerged as a major advance of modern medicine, providing high-quality life years to patients with end-stage renal disease (ESRD) [1, 2]. The prevalence of end-stage renal disease requiring transplantation in India is estimated to be between 151 and 232 per million population [3]. Post-transplant monitoring of the transplanted kidney is based on physical examination, urine volume, the assessment of albuminuria or proteinuria, serum creatinine, and glomerular filtration rate (GFR) estimation based on serum creatinine [4]. Of these multiple investigations, serum creatinine and urine analysis is one of the most widely used and accepted tool to asses graft dysfunction [3]. Urine examination, known as "Uroscopy" in ancient time was considered as the mirror of medicine for several thousands of years. The physicians felt they could view the body's inner workings and get the insight of the disease process by urine examination [5]. Urine examination aids diagnosis as well as management of both native as well as allograft kidney diseases [6].

Specific patterns in urinalysis provide information about graft function as well as renal diseases that can influence graft function [7]. It is a readily accessible, non-invasive tool, can be repeated anytime, cost effective as well as better tolerated than an invasive renal allograft biopsy. There are various causes for graft dysfunction, and these could be either acute or late. Urine analysis can help in diagnosis, follow-up and as well help in determining the graft outcome. Urinary abnormalities, such as hematuria or casts, are also useful in detecting and diagnosing allograft dysfunction [8, 9].

1.1 Causes of graft dysfunction

Before discussing about the role of urinalysis, it is important to determine the reasons for renal allograft dysfunction [9, 10]. Renal allograft dysfunction may be acute or late, the causes can broadly be classified as immunological or non-immunological. The immunological causes are usually acute and chronic rejections. The non-immunological causes include recurrence of a native disease, infections (bacterial, viral or fungal), acute tubular injury, drug toxicity, vascular complications, etc. [10]

Various parameters have been analyzed in urine of renal transplant recipients. These include determination of urine volume, urine osmolality, protein, glucose, blood and leucocytes. We conducted a pilot study in 310 renal transplant recipients who underwent renal allograft biopsy over a period of one year, where we analyzed the corresponding urinary findings which were compared with the morphological findings on renal allograft biopsy.

2. Urine osmolality

Osmolality marks the renal concentrating power, which depends on tubular function of the nephrons. Mazloum et al. in their study observed that altered osmoregulation performance, three months after transplantation is independently associated with allograft loss as well as reduced mGFR at 12 months [11]. When the graft suffers an ischemic lesion, the osmolality is lower as compared to that of a healthy kidney [12]. When we analyzed our set of patients, we found that the mean osmolality for patients with morphological evidence of rejection on RAB was 322.7 ± 141.3 mOsmol/l. This value was high as compared to patients having biopsy that were unremarkable for any immune or non-immune injury (mean urine osmolality: 116.2 ± 75.2 mOsmol/l). The osmolality of patients with biopsy features of acute tubular injury was 210 ± 82.2 mOsmol/l. Overall we recorded a higher value for urine osmolality in patients having acute rejection as compared to acute tubular injury or an unremarkable graft morphology.

Similar findings were also reported by Jenni et al. The receiver operator curve for osmolaluria to predict a rejection in the first 14 postoperative days showed an AUC (area under the curve) of 0.816 on day 2. The same study observed that if osmolaluria falls below 600 mOsmol/l, sensitivity and specificity for prediction of rejection is 66.7% and 89.5%, respectively [7]. Otto Schuck et al. examined early-morning urine osmolality in 104 transplant recipients (aged 21–76 years) and compared with findings of chronic renal allograft nephropathy by studying changes of interstitial fibrosis and tubular atrophy on biopsy. They postulated that the concentrating capacity of the graft kidney is decreased, however they did not report a significant correlation between concentrating function and tubulointerstitial histology findings with a mean urine osmolality of 384 ± 120 mOsmol/l [13]. In our patients with chronic renal allograft nephropathy the mean osmolality was found to be 282.4 ± 137.1 mOsmol/L. In biopsies with morphological features of interstitial fibrosis and tubular atrophy the mean urine osmolality was 242.2 ± 114.4 mOsmol/l. We conclude that alone urine osmolality might not be a good variable for diagnosis. The values need to be interpreted with respect to clinical features as well as taking other findings in considerations.

3. Proteinuria

Proteinuria (including albuminuria) is an independent factor implicated in kidney damage in native as well as kidney allografts [14]. Recommendations are to perform urinalysis and urinary protein excretion to be assessed regularly in the post-transplant period. Most of the studies recommend that these investigations need to be performed at least every 2 to 3 months during the first post-transplant year and annually henceforth [8]. Many unique proteins, peptides, and other substances are excreted in urine in the patients who undergo renal transplant which could be useful to predict the outcome of the renal allograft [15, 16]. It is estimated that proteinuria is a common finding in post-transplant patients, the incidence being more than 40% kidney transplant per year. Various studies have found that even if proteinuria is low (<500 mg/day), there is still significant reduction in the graft function and reduced patient survival [17]. Even late onset proteinuria in post-transplant patients has been found to be associated with reduced graft and patient survival [18]. Proteinuria in the first year of transplant appears to be multi-factorial. Common causes of proteinuria implicated are residual proteinuria, glomerular diseases, effects of anti-HLA class II antibodies and drugs like mTOR inhibitors, tubulointerstitial disease of the graft, nephrosclerosis, renal vein thrombosis and reflux nephropathy [7, 17]. Causes for late onset proteinuria in renal transplant patients include: relapse or de novo glomerulonephritis, transplant glomerulopathy and chronic rejections. A proteinuria of >0.5 g/l and > 0.8 g/l have found to have a specificity of 80% and 90%, respectively, regarding prediction of rejection [7]. Studies have shown pre-transplant proteinuria (even of nephrotic range) considerable reduces in the first weeks, once a normal functioning kidney is transplanted [7, 17]. This happens due to reduction in the blood flow which occurs in native kidneys after transplant, if the graft is functioning normally. In a patient with poor graft function, the blood flow of native kidneys is maintained, which is the cause for persistent proteinuria in such patients. For patients with a normal functioning graft, the presence of proteinuria above 3000 mg/day, three weeks after the transplant should raise a suspicion for presence of a glomerular disease. This could either be a de novo or a recurrence of a primary glomerulonephritis in the graft.

Many studies have studied the causes for post-transplant proteinuria. Among the commonly used immunosuppressive agents, only Sirolimus has been implicated in development of post- transplantation proteinuria [19]. One of the studies documented that 58% of transplant patients with proteinuria (150 mg/day) did demonstrate transplant-specific lesions (allograft nephropathy, transplant glomerulopathy, or acute rejection) on biopsy as compared to 11% of patients that showed morphological evidence of glomerulonephritis on biopsy [20]. Shamseddin et al. in his meta-analysis stated that allograft nephropathy was documented in 8–54% of patients (average: 32%). Transplant glomerulopathy ranged from 0 to 39% (average: 17%) with an average prevalence of 37% as compared to glomerular disease [21].

Various methods have been implicated in estimation of urinary protein. Of all the methods available, urine dipstick testing is highly specific and most commonly used method used in most of the laboratories. Despite of false-positive or false-negative results that can be obtained in some situations, it is still the most preferred screening method for proteinuria. As urine dip-stick is not as sensitive as quantitative methods, a twenty-four-hour urine protein excretion stands as the gold standard for quantitative protein assessment. In cases where a twenty-four hour urine collection is problematic, urinary protein/creatinine (mg/mg) ratio can be assessed in a 'spot' urine. A UPCR acts as an excellent surrogate and is shown to have an excellent correlation with the protein content of a twenty-four-hour urine collection [22].

In our study the mean 24-hour urinary proteinuria was highest in cases which presented with recurrence of the native disease (4.9 ± 2.31 g) followed by patients with biopsies showing chronic allograft nephropathy (2.69 ± 1.96 g). Proteinuria was insignificant in biopsies with acute rejection (0.5 ± 1.46 g). Of the recurrent diseases maximum proteinuria was observed in biopsies showing focal and segmental glomerulosclerosis (5.7 ± 3.8 g), followed by those with IgA nephropathy (4.4 ± 3.6 g) and membranoproliferative glomerulonephritis (4.5 ± 1.7 g). Thus evaluation by 24-hour urine protein does help in diagnosis of recurrent diseases as well as chronic allograft nephropathy.

4. Glucosuria

Recurrence of diabetic nephropathy in renal allograft and post-transplant diabetes mellitus are the main reasons for glycosuria. Multiple factors come into play for the above stated diseases. These include transplant done in an old aged patient, high body mass index, presence of a family history of diabetes, use of immunosuppressive reagents (Prednisone, Tacrolimus) and concomitant history of hypertension. Other risk factors include polycystic kidney disease, episode of immune injury (acute rejection), hepatitis B virus infection and hepatitis C virus infection. However the KDIGO guidelines recommend determination of blood glucose levels and glycosylated hemoglobin for diagnosis of diabetes, the role for the measurement of glucosuria after renal transplantation is limited [7, 23]. In our study of one year, we did not come across any case of glycosuria or post-transplant new onset diabetic nephropathy.

5. Hematuria

Presence of at least five red blood cells/high power field (hpf) in three of three consecutive centrifuged specimens obtained at least seven days apart is defined as hematuria [24]. Haematuria may be present in 0.7–3% of the general population, and has a much higher prevalence in patients undergoing renal transplant. Hematuria, like proteinuria has been implicated as one of the factors for graft loss [25]. Increased bleeding tendency in renal allograft recipients could be possibly due to preexisting states of postrenal transplant patients, the use of antiplatelet agents for cardiovascular disease and platelet dysfunction. Additionally, post-transplant patients are susceptible to anemia which accentuates bleeding diathesis. This usually occurs as the circulating red blood cells displace platelets towards the vessel wall thus leading to contact with the subendothelial tissue at the site of injury. Also red blood cells release adenosine diphosphate which inactivates prostacyclin and enhances platelet function [25, 26]. Although mechanisms of hematuria are many, following causes are main causes for hematuria in renal transplant patients:

5.1 Infections

Immunosuppressants are mainstay for graft stability, however use of these agents predisposes patients to urinary tract infections, which can be heralded by the sign of haematuria. Rivera-Sanchez conducted a prospective study on post-renal transplant patients with hematuria. They reported nearly 37% of the renal transplant recipients with hematuria have urinary tract infection, of which 13.4% had history of recurrent infections [27]. Certain predisposing factors have been implicated in causing recurrent acute graft pyelonephritis. These include presence of anatomical abnormalities like strictures at the ureterovesical junction or neurogenic bladder. Vesicoureteral reflux in these patients also contribute to recurrent infections [24]. As these patients are immunosuppressed, a higher index of suspicion for mycobacterial, fungal, and viral infection has to be kept in mind. Hematuria can occur secondary to cystitis, sparing the kidneys and can be associated with bacteria, fungus or viruses. Fungal organisms associated with hemorrhagic cystitis include *Candida albicans*, Cryptococcus, Aspergillus fumigates and mucormycosis whereas viruses implicated include BK virus, adenovirus, Cytomegalovirus, and herpes virus [28, 29].

5.2 Malignancy

Patients undergoing renal transplant are at risk of developing certain malignancies, in particular those cancers that are associated with viral infections. Common viruses include human papillomavirus (HPV) for cutaneous malignancies and Epstein–Barr virus (EBV) which are associated with post-transplant lymphoproliferative diseases.

Incidence of urological malignancies in these patients is less common. However some malignancies that can occur in these patients and present as hematuria include, renal cell carcinoma and cancers of the urinary bladder. Risk factors implicated in development of renal cell carcinoma are: prior history of renal cell carcinoma, polycystic kidney disease (PKD), duration of dialysis pre-transplant and tuberous sclerosis [30]. Larcom et al. showed that there is an estimated twofold increase for development of prostate carcinoma in the first 3 years after transplantation [31].

5.3 Rejections

Chronic rejection of the transplanted kidney typically presents with microscopic haematuria. Isolated case reports of patients with rejection presenting with gross haematuria have been documented [32].

5.4 Disease recurrences

Haematuria is a common manifestation of recurrence of glomerulonephritis. Those glomerulonephritis which present with a primarily nephritic picture present with hematuria predominantly. These commonly include Goodpasture's syndrome, systemic lupus erythematosus, and Ig A nephropathy. Acute syndromes that present with hematuria and lead to acute progressive renal failure with proteinuria and anemia include anti-neutrophil cytoplasmic autoantibodies (ANCA) and anti-glomerular basement membrane (GBM) glomerulonephritis [33].

Another remote cause for hematuria is development of a pseudoaneurysm in renal transplant recipient. A pseudoaneurysm is defined as arterial dilation accompanied with disruption of the one or more layers of the arterial wall. This lesion may be present at the site of puncture as a complication of procedures like arterial catheterization or as a complication of percutaneous nephrolithotomy (PCN). This procedure is done in a native or a transplanted kidney following a urinary tract obstruction and an infected hydronephrosis. Other reasons for doing a PCN include: urinary leakage, to remove calculi or a foreign body, chemotherapy and for urinary diversion due to hemorrhagic cystitis [34].

In our pilot study we observed hematuria in 35 (11.2%) patients. Of these 15 (4.8%) of a total 43 patients with active antibody mediated rejection (AMR) presented with hematuria, i.e. 34.8% patients with active AMR showed RBCs in their urine. Of 15 (4.8%) patients having recurrent glomerulonephritis, 9 (60%) presented with hematuria, five had IgA nephropathy and two each of C3 glomerulopathy and systemic lupus nephritis. None of the patients with acute tubular injury or chronic rejections or cellular rejection pr with patients with biopsy reported as unremarkable presented with hematuria. Thus, hematuria if present does indicate a disease process of graft.

5.5 Urinary tract infection (UTI)

Patients undergoing renal transplant have a suppressed immune response and hence have poor resistance to infection. Thus, infections in these group of patients is quite a common leading to morbidity and mortality post-transplantation [35]. Infections are the second most common cause for causing death in patients with renal transplant. The most common cause for predisposition of these patients to infection is that they are immunocompromised. Infection of the urinary tract is the most common infection affecting these subsets of patients, with an estimated incidence between 10 and 98% and is implicated for a longer hospital stay as well as increased health care cost [36–38].

Urine examination plays an indispensable role in diagnosis of urinary tract infection. Significant quantitative bacterial count (of ≥105 CFU/mL) in an appropriately collected urine sample aids the diagnosis of UTI in patients showing signs and symptoms of urinary tract infection [37]. Urinalysis in adjunct with urine culture studies are essential in determination of the causative organism of pyuria [39]. Presence of leucocytes in urine is an indicator of acute pyelonephritis and urinary tract infection [36, 37].

UTI can have enormous consequences on the lives of kidney recipients. For instance, it is the most common source of bloodstream infection among recipients, especially when it occurs during the first three months after transplantation [40]. Evaluations of UTI effects on renal parenchyma have shown how infections of the urinary system may result in prolonged inflammation and potential renal scarring [40, 41], which can lead to impaired renal function [42].

6. Role of novel biomarkers in renal transplant recipients

With advances in the field of renal transplantation, newer modalities for monitoring graft function have been developed. Determination of novel biomarkers in urine, plasma, serum and tissue have been implicated in monitoring renal allograft function. According to WHO, a novel biomarker is defined as a "alteration occurring at cellular, biochemical or molecular level in cells, tissues or body fluid which can be measured and evaluated to indicate the normal biological or a pathogenic processes, or a pharmacological response to a therapeutic intervention [43, 44]. Serum creatinine level, is the most commonly used biochemical parameter to assess the renal allograft function, but is not an affective marker to detect early renal dysfunction. This happens as creatinine concentration in serum is greatly influenced even by various non-renal factors (factors influencing serum creatinine levels: body weight, race, age, gender, total body volume, drugs, muscle metabolism, protein intake) [4, 43]. Additionally, it is not able to predict or evaluate the progression of chronic injury and making it a non-specific or non-predictive marker for graft dysfunction. Alternatively, this makes the histological examination through renal allograft biopsy the gold standard to determine the immunological or non-immunological cause for graft dysfunction [4, 11]. Therefore, these biomarkers, can be used for diagnosis of patients with a disease or an abnormal organ function and also to know the severity and prognosis of a disease, as well as monitor response to a medical procedure [4]. Thus, it is predicted that estimation of these novel biomarkers could possibly help in early recognition of allograft disease as well as help in monitoring disease activity. In addition to this, it is predicted that the novel marker estimation would optimizing the need for an invasive biopsy [45–47].

However, biopsy being an invasive procedure, may not be straightforward to perform and can be complicated by major bleeding. Other drawbacks associated are: risk of potential sampling errors, the inter-observer variability in assigning Banff scores and associated cost of the procedure. Hence it is not only impractical, it is also cumbersome and economically not feasible to monitor graft function by renal biopsy. Urine, on the other hand are readily available and direct product of the allograft and have minimal influence from systemic inflammation, making it a more desirable source for biomarkers [48].

An ideal biomarker is supposed to have certain characteristics. These include readily availability, accuracy, low cost, should be easy to standardized, produce repeatable results and be non-invasive. Overall such a biomarker should be useful to reduce the necessity for performing a renal allograft biopsy and help the clinician for early management [43, 44, 48].

6.1 Classification of novel biomarkers for renal allografts

Biomarkers used to monitor renal allografts can be grouped under two broad headings [44]:

- Immunologic biomarkers: Immunologic biomarkers are those characterizing immune dysfunction ranging from subclinical to overt rejection. These include following:

- Chemokines: Cystine-X-Cystine (C-X-C) motif chemokines 9 and 10, Plasma-derived fractalkine, IFN-γ, and interferon gamma-induced protein 10, cluster of differentiation thirty (CD30).

- Free micro ribonucleic acid: specific serum microRNAs miR-15B, miR-103A, and miR-106A, miR-223-3p, miR-424-3p, miR-145-5p.

- Leukocyte subclasses: donor-reactive memory B cells (mBCs), Donor-specific memory CD4 T cells.
- Gene expression profiles: Kidney Solid Organ Response Test (17 gene set), TruGraf® Molecular diagnostic test.
- Donor-derived cell-free deoxyribonucleic acid:
- Non-immunological biomarkers: Biomarkers that demonstrate adverse transplant outcomes, where immune dysfunction is not the only sole aberration implicated in the disease process, e.g., delayed graft function, cardiovascular events, infection, malignancy.
- Graft quality: The first and foremost important step in kidney transplantation is appropriate allocation of the organs and to predict the future outcome of transplanted organ. The biomarkers in this category include neutrophil gelatinase-associated lipocalin (NGAL) and liver fatty acid binding protein, KIM-1.
- Delayed graft function: It's a type of acute kidney injury, occurring in the first week after transplantation making renal replacement therapy essential for management. This group includes determination of NGAL.

6.2 Neutrophil gelatinase-associated lipocalin (NGAL) (Aka: uterocalin/lipocalin-2, 24p3/siderocalin)

This molecule is a member of lipocalin superfamily with molecular weight of is a 21 kD [49]. NGAL is secreted by neutrophils, acting as an acute-phase proteins [44]. First discovered as a complex protein with human neutrophil gelatinase in 1993 [49]. NGAL molecule is found in 3 isoforms: monomeric (25 kDa), dimeric (45 kDa), and as heterodimeric (135 kDa—complexed with gelatinase) [49]. The gene for this protein is located on chromosome 9 and this molecule is expressed in renal, liver, endothelial, smooth muscle cells, neurons, and cells of immune system (macrophages and dendritic cells) [50–52]. NGAL molecule expresses its action via a primary ligand, siderophore and metalloproteinase 9 (MMP-9) and is present in plasma as well as urine [4, 49]. Why is NGAL considered to be a biomarker of choice? The reason is that this biomarker is quite efficient and accurate in detecting kidney injury, very early in the post-transplant period. It is observed that there occurs a rapid rise of NGAL in urine, which is detectable even within few hours after the initial insult, whereas rise in serum creatinine occurs hours later [53]. Following AKI, the glomerular filtration rate (GFR) is also reduced which in turn causes the levels of NGAL to rise. A study showed that in patients with acute kidney injury, the levels of NGAL in blood and urine increase by 300-fold (0.1–30 μg/ml) and 1000-fold (0.04–40 mg/ml), respectively [52]. In severe cases of acute tubular injury large quantities of NGAL is excreted into urine, reaching almost up to 1000-fold. This happens due to induction of NGAL mRNA and protein in the renal epithelium as this molecule is expressed in the renal epithelium. Many studies have postulated that patients with higher urinary NGAL values in the early posttransplant phases are more prone to develop delayed graft dysfunction [53]. It has been observed that increase in serum creatinine happens several hours after renal cell destruction, but increase in urine/blood levels of NGAL can be observed as early as two hours of inception of injury. Thus, it is suggested that NGAL can be used to assess transplant status as early as a few hours post-transplantation [4].

6.3 Kidney injury molecule: 1 (KIM-1)

This protein is a type-1 transmembrane glycoprotein. KIM-1 comprises of two domains, viz.: six-cysteine immunoglobulin-like domain and a mucin domain (extracellular) [54]. KIM-1 also known as HAVCR/TIM-1 is a protein of 104 kD and the gene for this protein is located on chromosome 5q33.2 [4, 55]. KIM-1 (designated as Kim-1 in rodents, KIM-1 in humans) mRNA was identified using techniques of representational difference analysis (which is a PCR-based technique). This technique, which was carried out to find genes, the expression of which was found to be markedly upregulated 24–48 hours after ischaemia in the rat [56]. KIM-1 is expressed in the kidney, liver, and spleen and uninjured kidney tissue. Urine expresses very low or undetectable levels of KIM-1. Studies have shown that KIM-1 plays different roles via various molecular targets in immune diseases and kidney injury. This molecule is expressed on the apical membrane surface of proximal tubular epithelial cells of the kidney (in the S3 segment) and readily responds to hypoxia and renal tubular injury. The extracellular domain of KIM-1 molecule is a quantitative marker of kidney injury and is detached by metalloproteinases and then secreted into the urine. KIM-1 is also an important marker for kidney transplant rejection [52–55]. Various studies including one by Jin et al. reported that serum KIM-1 might be a marker for the prediction of early kidney transplant rejection. They also predicted that this molecule could possibly be helpful in monitoring renal graft function in transplant recipients, and thus might contribute in early diagnosis of organ rejection [57].

6.4 C-X-C motif chemokine 10 (CXCL-10)

This molecule is an interferon-γ-inducible protein-10 (IP-10), a chemokine belonging to the CXC subfamily. This molecule consists of two cysteines that are located at the N-terminus. These two cysteines are separated by a single amino acid which can be variable [58]. The gene for this protein is located on chromosome 4. This chemokine is excreted from all the leukocytes, viz. neutrophils, eosinophils, monocytes and epithelial, endothelial, as well as stromal cells and keratinocytes. The chemokine is secreted as a response to several proinflammatory factors, like interferon γ (IFN γ) [58, 59]. CXCL-10 is secreted by leukocytes in the transplanted kidney and is a marker for inflammation. According to the observations of Elkman et al. CXCL9 and CXCL10, which are induced by IFNγ are supposedly to be the most studied as well as promising protein biomarkers for predicting acute renal rejection. Both CXCL9 and CXCL10 bind with CXCR3, that are expressed on activated T-cell which in turn recruit T-cells to the inflammatory site [45]. Schaub et al. demonstrated that the sensitivity and specificity of urinary CXCL-10 (uCXCL-10) exceeded those of serum creatinine levels. Various studies have been performed to determine the role of CXCL10 molecule in allogenic kidney transplant rejection. Study by Ciftci et al. which was performed on living donor related transplant recipients to assess the efficacy of CXCL10, showed that urine levels of CXCL-10 correlates well with serum creatinine level is patients having acute cellular rejection [60–62]. On the other hand, Rabant et al. studied 244 renal allotransplant recipients and monitored urinary CXCL-10 and serum creatinine levels. They further determined the ratio of CXCL10 and serum creatinine and proposed that the ratio can effectively determine the risk of antibody-dependent transplant rejection [63].

Blydt-Hansen et al. also reported similar observation for the CXCL-10 to creatinine ratio in pediatric renal transplant recipients and concluded CXCL-10 to be a promising biomarker of acute cellular rejection [64]. Matz et al. in his study reported that CXCL-10 chemokine levels may predict the development of acute cell-type rejection [65]. Watson et al. demonstrated that high pretransplant serum CXCL-10 levels may indicate a high risk of severe rejection and transplant failure and it would be appropriate to determine the CXCL-10 levels pre-transplantation [66]. Jackson et al. found that urine CXCL-10 levels can increase in acute transplant rejection as well as in patients suffering from polyoma virus nephropathy, however this chemokine cannot be used to differentiate between these two conditions [67].

6.5 Calreticulin (CRT)

CRT is a major calcium 2+ (Ca2+) binding (storage) protein. This protein is present in the lumen of the endoplasmic reticulum with a molecular weight of 46 kDa, having 400 amino acid residues. This protein is basically a major Ca2+ binding chaperon. Calreticulin has three distinct structural domains: the amino-terminal N-domain, middle P-domain, and the terminal carboxyl-C-domain along with a cleavable amino acid signal sequence. This amino acid signal sequence is present at the beginning of the N-terminal, which helps in directing CRT to the endoplasmic reticulum. The C-terminal functions for ER retention/retrieval signal. Two main functions have been implicated to this protein in the ER: One as a chaperon and other as a Ca2+ binding and storage protein. It can be identified at several other sub-cellular locations like cell surface, cytoplasm, and the extracellular matrix [68].

6.6 Cystatin C (CysC)

CysC is an endogenous proteinase inhibitor with a molecular weight of ~13.4 kD. This molecule is a member of cystatin superfamily of cysteine protease inhibitors. The main function of the protein is to inhibit cathepsins, namely cathepsin L, B, and H [69, 70]. CysC is composed of polypeptide chain having 120 amino acids and the chromosome 20 harbors the gene for this protein [71]. CysC has a role in intracellular catabolism of proteins and peptides. Another advantage of this protein is that concentration of CysC does not depend on factors like gender, age, or muscle mass, making it more suitable to determine the dynamics of GFR changes as compared to serum creatinine [72]. Krishnamurthy et al. concluded CysC as an additional diagnostic parameter in assessing the function of a transplanted organ, which additionally might be helpful and serve to tailor immunosuppressive treatment [73]. Changes in the glomerular filtration rate secondary to a deteriorating transplant function and thus an increased risk of rejection, can be detected by the determination of cystatin C according to, according to Taghizadeh Afshari et al. Study by A. Taghizadeh-Afshari showed that at 14 days post-transplant, levels of CysC exceeds the sensitivity and specificity of serum creatinine [74]. Similar observations were also made by Le Bricon et al. According to him CysC is a more accurate marker than serum creatinine. He additionally postulated role of Cystatin C in assessing the toxic effects of treatment [75].

6.7 Osteopontin (OPN):0020

Osteopontin, also known as bone sialoprotein 1 (BSP-1) or secreted phosphoprotein 1 (SPP1) and also as early T-lymphocyte activation-1 (ETA-1). This protein is an extracellular matrix protein with a molecular weight of approximately 35 kD. It is composed of a polypeptide chain comprising of 314 amino acids. The polypeptide chain contains sequence of arginine-glycine-asparagine binding integrin [76–78]. This molecule is encoded by a single-copy gene which is mapped on the human chromosome 4 (4q13). This molecule is expressed on intestinal epithelial cells, bone, kidney, and immune cells, such as macrophages, dendritic cells, and the T lymphocytes [79, 80]. The serum osteopontin concentration in a normal individual is estimated to be around 23.56 ng/ml [80]. Osteopontin, in kidney, is produced at distal part of nephron. The function of this molecule is implicated in formation of renal vessels [81, 82].

6.8 Clusterin (CLU)

CLU is also called as apolipoprotein J (CLU). It is a glycosylated protein and is composed of two chains, the α-chain and β-chain. These both are linked via disulfide bonds and in human body it is present in two isoforms – secretory type and nuclear type. The mass of the secretory type is 80 kD, and is implicated in removing residues formed after apoptosis. The nuclear type isoform is 50 kD and has its role in DNA repair. The gene encoding for this protein is located on chromosome 8. Clusterin molecule has a role in apoptosis as well as in antiapoptotic pathway. CLU in human body is present in various organs, including kidney and is also detected in all biological fluids. The physiological concentrations of CLU in serum range from 35 to 105 μg/ml. In kidney, this molecule is present in the tubules and has numerous antiapoptotic functions, by mediating cell protection, recycling of lipids, attachment and aggregation of cells. Although the function or utility of CLU in renal transplant rejection is yet to be analyzed [83–85].

7. Conclusion

Multiple causes can affect the functioning of the renal allograft, and there are multiple modalities that are recommended in evaluation of the renal transplant. In the present era where most of the investigations fall under the category of molecular tests and genetics, immunohistochemistry, cytogenetics etc., urine examination still plays an indispensable role in management of the renal allograft. Overall certain parameters like urine osmolality, proteinuria, hematuria and urine microscopy along with the newer molecules (biomarkers) are a hit and help in monitoring of the renal allograft.

Author details

Lovelesh K. Nigam
Laboratory Medicine, Department of Pathology, Transfusion Services and Immunohematology, G.R. Doshi and K.M. Mehta Institute of Kidney Diseases and Research Centre and Dr. H.L. Trivedi Institute of Transplantation Sciences, Ahmedabad, India

*Address all correspondence to: drloveleshnigam@gmail.com

References

[1] Garcia GG, Harden P, Chapman J. The global role of kidney transplantation. Kidney & Blood Pressure Research. 2012;**35**:299-304. DOI: 10.1159/000337044

[2] Abecassis M, Bartlett ST, Collins AJ, Davis CL, Delmonico FL, Friedewald JJ, et al. Kidney transplantation as primary therapy for end-stage renal disease: A National Kidney Foundation/kidney disease outcomes quality initiative (NKF/KDOQITM) conference. Clinical Journal of the American Society of Nephrology. 2008;**3**(2):471-480. DOI: 10.2215/CJN.05021107

[3] Shroff S. Current trends in kidney transplantation in India. Indian Journal of Urology. 2016;**32**(3):173-174. DOI: 10.4103/0970-1591.185092

[4] Rogulska K, Wojciechowska-Koszko I, Dołęgowska B, Kwiatkowska E, Roszkowska P, et al. The Most promising biomarkers of allogeneic kidney transplant rejection. Journal of Immunology Research; 2022. 18 pages. Article ID 6572338. DOI: 10.1155/2022/6572338

[5] Armstrong JA. Urinalysis in Western culture: A brief history. Kidney International. 2007;**71**:384-387

[6] Hashmi P, Ho C, Morgan S, Stephenson JR. Routine urinanalysis in renal transplant patients. Journal of Clinical Pathology. 1995;**48**:383-384

[7] Jenni F, Riethmüller S, Wüthrich RP. Significance of urine diagnostic tests after renal transplantation. Kidney & Blood Pressure Research. 2013;**37**:116-123. DOI: 10.1159/000350065

[8] Kidney Disease: Improving Global Outcomes (KDIGO) Transplant Work Group. KDIGO clinical practice guideline for the care of kidney transplant recipients. American Journal of Transplantation. 2009;**9**(Suppl. 3):S1-S155

[9] Kunthara MG, Sahay M, Hussain HI, Ismal K, Vali PS, Kavadi A, et al. Posttransplant renal allograft dysfunction – A retrospective observational study. Indian Journal of Transplantation. 2021;**15**:232-240

[10] Goldberg RJ, Weng FL, Kandula P. Acute and chronic allograft dysfunction in kidney transplant recipients. Medical Clinics of North America. May 2016;**100**(3):487-503. DOI: 10.1016/j.mcna.2016.01.002. PMID: 27095641

[11] Mazloum M, Jouffroy J, Brazier F, Legendre C, Neuraz A, Garcelon N, et al. Osmoregulation performance and kidney transplant outcome. Journal of the American Society of Nephrology. 2019;**30**(7):1282-1293. DOI: 10.1681/ASN.2018121269

[12] Zimmermann-Spinnler M. Urinlabor. Liestal CH: Medical Laboratory Consulting AG; 1991. pp. S41-S44

[13] Ondiej OS, Voska VL, Yladimir AJ, et al. Early morning urine osmolality in patients with chronic allograft nephropathy. Transplant International. 2004;**17**:270-271. DOI: 10.1007/s00147-004-0707-6

[14] Amer H, Filder ME, Myslak M, Morales P, Kremers WK, Larson TS, et al. Proteinuria after kidney transplantation, relationship to allograft histology and survival. American Journal of Transplantation. 2007;7(12):2748-2756. DOI: 10.1111/j.1600-6143.2007.02006.x

[15] Stevens LA, Coresh J, Greene T, et al. Assessing kidney function–measured

and estimated glomerular filtration rate. The New England Journal of Medicine. 2006;**354**:2473-2483

[16] Knoll GA. Proteinuria in kidney transplant recipients: Prevalence, prognosis, and evidence-based management. American Journal of Kidney Diseases. 2009;**54**(6):1131-1144

[17] Suárez Fernández ML, G-Cosío F. Causes and consequences of proteinuria following kidney transplantation. Nefrología. 2011;**31**(4):404-414. English, Spanish. DOI: 10.3265/Nefrologia.pre2011.May.10972

[18] Fernández-Fresnedo G, Plaza J, Sánchez-Plumed J, Sanz-Guajardo A, Palomar-Fontanet R, Arias M. Proteinuria: A new marker of long-term graft and patient survival in kidney transplantation. Nephrology, Dialysis, Transplantation. 2004;**19**:iii47-iii51

[19] Rangan GK. Sirolimus-associated proteinuria and renal dysfunction. Drug Safety. 2006;**29**(12):1153-1161. DOI:10.2165/00002018-200629120-00006

[20] Oblak M, Mlinšek G, Kojc N, Frelih M, Buturović-Ponikvar J, Arnol M. Spot urine protein excretion in the first year following kidney transplantation associates with allograft rejection phenotype at 1-year surveillance biopsies: An observational National-Cohort Study. Frontiers in Medicine (Lausanne). 2021;**8**:781195. DOI: 10.3389/fmed.2021.781195

[21] Khaled SM, Knoll Greg A. Posttransplantation proteinuria: An approach to diagnosis and management. Clinical Journal of the American Society of Nephrology. 2011;**6**(7):1786-1793. DOI: 10.2215/CJN.01310211

[22] Yang F, Shi JS, Gong SW, Xu XD, Le WB. An equation to estimate 24-hour total urine protein excretion rate in patients who underwent urine protein testing. BMC Nephrology. 2022;**23**(1):49. DOI: 10.1186/s12882-022-02673-2

[23] Xia M, Yang H, Tong X, Xie H, Cui F, Shuang W. Risk factors for new-onset diabetes mellitus after kidney transplantation: A systematic review and meta-analysis. Journal of Diabetes Investigation. 2021;**12**(1):109-122. DOI: 10.1111/jdi.13317

[24] Saleem MO, Hamawy K. Hematuria. [updated August 8, 2022]. In: StatPearls [Internet]. Treasure Island (FL): StatPearls Publishing; 2022 Available from: https://www.ncbi.nlm.nih.gov/books/NBK534213/

[25] Wang Z, Vathsala A, Tiong HY. Haematuria in postrenal transplant patients. BioMed Research International. 2015;**2015**:292034. DOI: 10.1155/2015/292034

[26] Trivedi HS, Lal SM, Gupta N, Ross R Jr. ATGAM associated coagulopathy in renal transplant patients: A report of two unusual cases. The International Journal of Artificial Organs. 1996;**19**(8):448-450

[27] Rivera-Sanchez R, Delgado-Ochoa D, Flores-Paz RR. Prospective study of urinary tract infection surveillance after kidney transplantation. BMC Infectious Diseases. 2010;**10**, Article 245. DOI: 10.1186/1471-2334-10-245

[28] Manikandan R, Kumar S, Dorairajan LN. Hemorrhagic cystitis: A challenge to the urologist. Indian Journal of Urology. 2010;**26**(2):159-166. DOI: 10.4103/0970-1591.65380

[29] Yagisawa T, Nakada T, Takahashi K, Toma H, Ota K, Yaguchi H. Acute Hemorrhagic cystitis caused by adenovirus after kidney transplantation. Urologia

Internationalis. 1995;**54**:142-146. DOI: 10.1159/000282708

[30] Schwarz A, Vatandaslar S, Merkel S, Haller H. Renal cell carcinoma in transplant recipients with acquired cystic kidney disease. Clinical Journal of the American Society of Nephrology. 2007;**2**(4):750-756

[31] Larcom RC Jr, Carter GH. Erythrocytes in urinary sediment: Identification and normal limits. With a note on the nature of granular casts. The Journal of Laboratory and Clinical Medicine. 1948;**33**(7):875-880

[32] Newman LB, Anderson EE, Schulman CC. Renal allograft rejection presenting with gross hematuria: Case report. Acta Urologica Belgica. 1972;**40**(4):825-829

[33] Nakamura T, Shirouzu T. Antibody-mediated rejection and recurrent primary disease: Two Main obstacles in abdominal kidney, liver, and pancreas transplants. Journal of Clinical Medicine. 2021;**10**(22):5417. DOI: 10.3390/jcm10225417

[34] Young M, Leslie SW. Percutaneous nephrostomy. [updated 2022 Nov 28]. In: StatPearls [Internet]. Treasure Island (FL): StatPearls Publishing; 2022 Available from: https://www.ncbi.nlm.nih.gov/books/NBK493205/

[35] Singh N, Limaye AP. Infections in solid-organ transplant recipients. In: Mandell, Douglas, and Bennett's Principles and Practice of Infectious Diseases. 2015. pp. 3440-3452. DOI: 10.1016/B978-1-4557-4801-3.00313-1. PMCID: PMC7151835

[36] Anastasopoulos NA, Duni A, Peschos D, Agnantis N, Dounousi E. The Spectrum of infectious diseases in kidney transplantation: A review of the classification, pathogens and clinical manifestations. Infectious Diseases in Kidney Transplantation. 2015;**29**:415-422

[37] Nigam LA, Vanikar AV, Patel RD, Kanodia KV, Suthar KS. Urinary Tract Infection in Renal Allograft Recipents. In: Tomas J, Daca A, Dębska-Ślizień MA, editors. London, UK: IntechOpen; [Internet]. 2018. DOI: 10.5772/intechopen.77171

[38] Olenski S, Scuderi C, Choo A, Bhagat Singh AK, Way M, Jeyaseelan L, et al. Urinary tract infections in renal transplant recipients at a quaternary care Centre in Australia. BMC Nephrology. 2019;**20**(1):479. DOI: 10.1186/s12882-019-1666-6

[39] Goldman JD, Julian K. Urinary tract infections in solid organ transplant recipients: Guidelines from the American Society of Transplantation infectious diseases Community of Practice. Clinical Transplantation. 2019;**33**(9):e13507. DOI: 10.1111/ctr.13507

[40] Memikoglu KO, Keven K, Sengul S, et al. Urinary tract infections following renal transplantation: A single-center experience. Transplantation Proceedings. 2007;**39**(10):3131-3347

[41] Ramsey DE, Finch WT, Birtch AG. Urinary tract infections in kidney transplant recipients. Archives of Surgery. 1979;**114**(9):1022-1025

[42] Ariza-Heredia EJ, Beam EN, Lesnick TG, Kremers WK, Cosio FG, Razonable RR. Urinary tract infections in kidney transplant recipients: Role of gender, urologic abnormalities, and antimicrobial prophylaxis. Annals of Transplantation. 2013;**18**:195-204. DOI: 10.12659/AOT.883901

[43] Wang H, Lin ZT, Yuan Y, Wu T. Urine biomarkers in renal allograft. Journal

of Translational Internal Medicine. 2016;**4**(3):109-113. DOI: 10.1515/jtim-2016-0032

[44] Swanson KJ, Aziz F, Garg N, Mohamed M, Mandelbrot D, Djamali A, et al. Role of novel biomarkers in kidney transplantation. World Journal of Transplantation. 2020;**10**(9):230-255 Available from: https://www.wjgnet.com/2220-3230/full/v10/i9/230.htm. DOI: 10.5500/wjt.v10.i9.230

[45] Eikmans M, Gielis EM, Ledeganck KJ, Yang J, Abramowicz D, Claas FFJ. Non-invasive biomarkers of acute rejection in kidney transplantation: Novel targets and strategies. Frontiers in Medicine (Lausanne). January 2019;**5**(8):358. DOI: 10.3389/fmed.2018.00358. PMID: 30671435; PMCID: PMC6331461

[46] Naesens M, Anglicheau D. Precision transplant medicine: Biomarkers to the rescue. Journal of the American Society of Nephrology. 2018;**29**:24-34

[47] Wiebe C, Ho J, Gibson IW, Rush DN, Nickerson PW. Carpe diem-time to transition from empiric to precision medicine in kidney transplantation. American Journal of Transplantation. 2018;**18**:1615-1625

[48] Guzzi F, Cirillo L, Buti E, Becherucci F, Errichiello C, Roperto RM, et al. Urinary biomarkers for diagnosis and prediction of acute kidney allograft rejection: A systematic review. International Journal of Molecular Sciences. 2020;**21**(18):6889. DOI: 10.3390/ijms21186889

[49] Ning M, Mao X, Niu Y, Tang B, Shen H. Usefulness and limitations of neutrophil gelatinase-associated lipocalin in the assessment of kidney disease. The Journal of Laboratory and Precision Medicine (JLPM). 2018;**3**(1). DOI: 10.21037/jlpm.20

[50] Al-Refai AA, Tayel SI, Ragheb A, et al. Urinary neutrophil gelatinase associated lipocalin as a marker of tubular damage in type 2 diabetic patients with and without albuminuria. Open Journal of Nephrology. 2014;**4**(1):37-46

[51] Szumilas D, Wojnar J, Chudek J. Neutrophil gelatinase-associated lipocalin as a marker of acute renal failure in cancer patients treated with cisplatin. Nowotwory. Journal of Oncology. 2016;**66**(2):160-166

[52] Beker B, Corleto M, Fieiras C, Musso C. Novel acute kidney injury biomarkers: Their characteristics utility and concerns. International Urology and Nephrology. 2018;**50**(4):705-713

[53] Cappuccilli M, Capelli I, Comai G, Cianciolo G, La Manna G. Neutrophil gelatinase-associated Lipocalin as a biomarker of allograft function after renal transplantation: Evaluation of the current status and future insights. Artificial Organs. 2018;**42**(1):8-14. DOI: 10.1111/aor.13039

[54] Bailly V, Zhang Z, Meier W, Cate R, Sanicola M, Bonventre JV. Shedding of kidney injury molecule-1, a putative adhesion protein involved in renal regeneration. Journal of Biological Chemistry. 2002;**277**(42): 39739-39748

[55] Medić B, Rovčanin B, Basta Jovanović G, Radojević-Škodrić S, Prostran M. Kidney injury molecule-1 and cardiovascular diseases: From basic science to clinical practice. BioMed Research International. 2015;**2015**:854070. . DOI: 10.1155/2015/854070. PMID: 26697493; PMCID: PMC4677159

[56] Bonventre JV. Kidney injury molecule-1 (KIM-1): A urinary

biomarker and much more. Nephrology, Dialysis, Transplantation. 2009;**24**:3265-3268. DOI: 10.1093/ndt/gfp010

[57] Jin ZK, Tian P, Wang X, et al. Kidney injury molecule-1 and osteopontin: New markers for prediction of early kidney transplant rejection. Molecular Immunology. 2013;**54**(3-4):457-464

[58] Neville LF, Mathiak G, Bagasra O. The immunobiology of interferon-gamma inducible protein 10 KD (IP-10): A novel, pleiotropic member of the C-X-C chemokine superfamily. Cytokine & Growth Factor Reviews. 1997;**8**(3):207-219

[59] Zlotnik A, Yoshie O. Chemokines: A new classification system and their role in immunity. Immunity. 2000;**12**(2):121-127

[60] Liu M, Guo S, Hibbert J, et al. CXCL10/IP-10 in infectious diseases pathogenesis and potential therapeutic implications. Cytokine & Growth Factor Reviews. 2011;**22**(3):121-130

[61] Schaub S, Nickerson P, Rush D, et al. Urinary CXCL9 and CXCL10 levels correlate with the extent of subclinical tubulitis. American Journal of Transplantation. 2009;**9**(6):1347-1353

[62] Ciftci HS, Tefik T, Savran MK, et al. Urinary CXCL9 and CXCL10 levels and acute renal graft rejection. International Journal of Organ Transplantation Medicine. 2019;**10**(2):53-63

[63] Rabant M, Amrouche L, Lebreton X, et al. Urinary C-X-C motif chemokine 10 independently improves the noninvasive diagnosis of antibody-mediated kidney allograft rejection. Journal of the American Society of Nephrology. 2015;**26**(11):2840-2851

[64] Blydt-Hansen TD, Gibson IW, Gao A, Dufault B, Ho J. Elevated urinary CXCL10-to-creatinine ratio is associated with subclinical and clinical rejection in pediatric renal transplantation. Transplantation. 2015;**99**(4):797-804

[65] Matz M, Beyer J, Wunsch D, et al. Early post-transplant urinary IP-10 expression after kidney transplantation is predictive of short- and long-term graft function. Kidney International. 2006;**69**(9):1683-1690

[66] Watson D, Yang JYC, Sarwal RD, et al. A novel multibiomarker assay for non-invasive quantitative monitoring of kidney injury. Journal of Clinical Medicine. 2019;**8**(4):499

[67] Jackson JA, Kim E, Begley B, et al. Urinary chemokines CXCL9 and CXCL10 are noninvasive markers of renal allograft rejection and BK viral infection. American Journal of Transplantation. 2011;**11**(10):2228-2234

[68] Gawish RIAR, El Aggan HAM, Mahmoud SAH, et al. A novel biomarker of chronic allograft dysfunction in renal transplant recipients (serum calreticulin and CD47). The Egyptian Journal of Internal Medicine. 2020;**32**:19. DOI: 10.1186/s43162-020-00018-9

[69] Murty MSN, Sharma UK, Pandey VB, Kankare SB. Serum cystatin C as a marker of renal function in detection of early acute kidney injury. Indian Journal of Nephrology. 2013;**23**(3):180-183

[70] Cimerman N, Prebanda MT, Turk B, Popovič T, Dolenc I, Turk V. Interaction of cystatin C variants with papain and human cathepsins B, H and L. Journal of Enzyme Inhibition. 1999;**14**(2):167-174

[71] Mareš J, Stejskal D, Vavroušková J, Urbánek K, Herzig R, Hluštík P. Use of cystatin C determination in clinical diagnostics. Biomed Papers. 2003;**147**(2):177-180

[72] Chew JS, Saleem M, Florkowski CM, George PM. Cystatin C–a paradigm of evidence based laboratory medicine. The Clinical Biochemist Reviews. 2008;**29**(2):47

[73] Krishnamurthy N, Arumugasamy K, Anand U, Anand CV, Aruna V, Venu G. Serum cystatin C levels in renal transplant recipients. Indian Journal of Clinical Biochemistry. 2011;**26**(2):120-124

[74] Taghizadeh-Afshari A, Mohammadi-Fallah M, Alizadeh M, et al. Serum cystatin C versus creatinine in the assessment of allograft function in early periods of kidney transplantation. Journal of Renal Injury Prevention. 2017;**7**(1):11-15

[75] Le Bricon T, Thervet E, Benlakehal M, Bousquet B, Legendre C, Erlich D. Changes in plasma cystatin C 16 journal of immunology research after renal transplantation and acute rejection in adults. Clinical Chemistry. 1999;**45**(12):2243-2249

[76] Wai PY, Kuo PC. The role of osteopontin in tumor metastasis. Journal of Surgical Research. 2004;**121**(2):228-241

[77] Christensen B, Nielsen MS, Haselmann KF, Petersen TE, Sørensen ES. Post-translationally modified residues of native human osteopontin are located in clusters: Identification of 36 phosphorylation and five O-glycosylation sites and their biological implications. Biochemical Journal. 2005;**390**(Part 1):285-292

[78] Young MF, Kerr JM, Termine JD, et al. CDNA cloning, MRNA distribution and heterogeneity, chromosomal location, and RFLP analysis of human osteopontin (OPN). Genomics. 1990;**7**(4):491-502

[79] Brown LF, Berse B, Van de Water L, et al. Expression and distribution of osteopontin in human tissues: Widespread association with luminal epithelial surfaces. Molecular Biology of the Cell. 1992;**3**(10):1169-1180

[80] Reza S, Shaukat A, Arain TM, Riaz QS, Mahmud M. Expression of osteopontin in patients with thyroid dysfunction. PLoS One. 2013;**8**(2):e56533. DOI: 10.1371/journal.pone.0056533

[81] Hudkins KL, Giachelli CM, Cui Y, Couser WG, Johnson RJ, Alpers CE. Osteopontin expression in fetal and mature human kidney. Journal of the American Society of Nephrology. 1999;**10**(3):444-457

[82] Rogers SA, Padanilam BJ, Hruska KA, Giachelli CM, HammermanMR.Metanephricosteopontin regulates nephrogenesis in vitro. American Journal of Physiology Renal Physiology. 1997;**272**(4):469-476

[83] De Silva HV, Harmony JAK, Stuart WD, Gil CM, Robbins J. Apolipoprotein J: Structure and tissue distribution. Biochemistry. 1990;**29**(22):5380-5389

[84] Pajak B, Orzechowski A. Clusterin: The missing link in the calcium-dependent resistance of cancer cells to apoptogenic stimuli. Postepy Higieny I Medycyny Doswiadczalnej (Online). 2006;**60**:45-51

[85] Jenne DE, Tschopp J. Clusterin: The intriguing guises of a widely expressed glycoprotein. Trends in Biochemical Sciences. 1992;**17**(4):154-159

Chapter 5

Application of Urine Metabolomics as a Marker in Health and Disease

Abraham Joseph Pellissery, Poonam Gopika Vinayamohan, Leya Susan Viju, Divya Joseph and Kumar Venkitanarayanan

Abstract

Advances in metabolomics research have yielded an avenue for utilizing this laboratory-based modality as a platform for clinical diagnosis, identification of novel biomarkers, and longitudinally monitoring the health status of individuals from normal physiological and pathophysiological perspectives. This chapter provides insight on the application of urinalysis in health and disease from the standpoint of deciphering a larger span of metabolite and biomarker identification using metabolomics, specifically focusing on infectious diseases, oncology, metabolic, and inflammatory diseases in humans.

Keywords: urine metabolome, urinalysis, pre-analytical factors, cancer, infectious disease, inflammation, metabolic disease, renal disease

1. Introduction

Urinalysis or uroscopy is the science of disease diagnosis by means of observation and examination of the urine. Urinalysis has been considered as an adjunct of all laboratory tests applied for medical diagnosis by correlating with the symptoms exhibited by patients and is historically referenced as the first body fluid to be studied scientifically [1, 2]. Ancient medical literature from India and China have referenced the accumulation of ants and insects around sites of urination of certain individuals who had obviously suffered from diabetes. The science of uroscopy was advocated in 300 BC by Hippocrates and was considered as a popular testing modality to link his observations with the doctrine of the four humors, that is, the phlegm, blood, yellow bile, and black bile. During those times, analysis of urine color, consistency, transparency, odor, and the presence or absence of froth aided to make a general assessment of the balance of the four humors and possibly location of the disease within the body and overall prognosis [2]. Throughout the medieval and post-seventeenth century periods, medical literature had cited urinalysis as an important foundation for medical practice. Although medical practice during the mid-nineteenth century had done away with the practice of uroscopy due to the advancements in human medicine, urinalysis still prevails as an important foundation and a powerful tool for clinical diagnosis [3]. Urinalysis has been used to identify genetic diseases as well as diagnose pathophysiological processes by measuring abnormal urine constituents such as glucose, bile pigments, white blood cells, proteins, etc. In addition, the presumptive diagnosis of diseases affecting the urogenital system can be inferred through urinalysis [3–5]. This chapter describes the applications of urine metabolomics in defining the biomarkers of health and clinical disease states.

2. Metabolomics in clinical urinalysis

Urine is an easily accessible biological fluid for noninvasive collection of large volumes with the possibility of repeat sampling at different time points, as needed for monitoring health status [6]. Traditionally, urinalysis tests conducted in diagnostic laboratories measured only one or two metabolite components (e.g., glucose, ketone bodies, etc.) at a given time [7]. Also, the abnormal urinary constituents tested via traditional methods lack specificity and are noticeable in urine samples after tissue injury. Therefore, an ideal biomarker in urine should be highly sensitive and specific and should be capable of indicating an early phase of disease progression [8].

Since the 1970s, urinary metabolome analysis has facilitated in investigation of metabolic signatures or fingerprints of urinary metabolites during the disease process in the human body [4, 8, 9]. Metabolomics is defined as the systemic identification and quantification of all metabolites in a given organism or biological sample [10]. Since metabolites generated in an organism are a result of several gene-level (host-dependent, genetic factors) and environmental-level interactions, the general metabolome, which includes the sum of all the metabolites in an organism, can serve as a critical biomarker analyte fingerprint for the health status of an individual's phenotype. Emerging technologies based on mass spectrometry (MS) and nuclear magnetic resonance spectrometry (NMR) enable the monitoring of hundreds of metabolites from tissues or body fluids. Metabolites change rapidly in response to physiological alterations, thus they act as the first-line chemical reporters of abnormal or disease phenotypes. Current advancements in high-resolution metabolomics platforms capable of detecting hundreds of low-molecular-weight metabolites in tissues and body fluids have evolved as a powerful biomarker analysis tool. The datasets generated from clinical trials and research studies curate for clinical databases that support diagnosis and therapeutic assessment of several disease states [7]. However, these datasets require standardization and validation to create a clinical reference guide that is applicable for any biofluid, as well as FDA approval for utilizing this platform for clinical diagnostic purposes [11].

3. Sample collection considerations for urine metabolomics

Urine metabolome has aided in the examination of metabolic consequence correlating to disease, nutritional status, and environmental toxicity since excreted urine contains endogenous and exogenous metabolites, thereby providing a key biomarker fingerprint to diagnose, monitor, or predict for any pathophysiological condition [12]. More than 3100 metabolites have been characterized in human urine, and the list is expected to increase as more and more low-concentration metabolites are being characterized [9]. With the intended application of urine samples for biomedical research or clinical diagnosis, pre-analytical factors such as collection methods and preprocessing, transport and storage, freeze-thaw cycles, and sample normalization are taken into consideration when processing metabolomic analysis [13]. Standardization of pre-analytical process is critical for minimizing inter-sample variability issues and maintaining the metabolic integrity of samples so that the metabolomic profile accurately reflects the *in vivo* biochemical status of the patient [13].

Generally, three kinds of collection modalities are employed for metabolomic studies involving urine samples: (a) first-morning void (b) spot urine samples, and (c) 24 h urine collection. The first-morning void urine samples are preferred since the overnight fast period helps to reduce the effect of any medication or the meal consumed from the previous day. Spot urine samples are the preferred sample type for dietary or pharmaceutical intervention studies and are usually collected during the daytime. However, pooled urine void samples during a 24 h duration reduce the influence of circadian cycle variation when compared to first void or spot urine samples [13].

Urine samples held at room temperature for short periods of time can lead to rapid degradation of metabolites. Considering the storage requirements of urine samples, it is optimal to freeze samples as soon as possible. Generally, while conducting clinical metabolomic studies, samples are refrigerated in autosamplers of MS and NMR instruments for time spans from hours to days. Ideally, it has been indicated by researchers that keeping samples at 4°C for 48 h or less does not significantly affect the urinary metabolome [9]. Although it would be prudent to minimize multiple freezing and thawing of urine samples, up to 9 freeze-thaw cycles are considered amenable for urine samples utilized for metabolomic studies. For long-term storage of up to 6 months or more, temperatures between −20 and −80°C are recommended. Another concern with urine collection and storage is bacterial contamination, which can be curtailed by collecting mid-stream urine and subsequently adding antibacterial agents such as sodium azide or sodium fluoride [9]. As an alternative, storage of samples at −80°C over the use of antibacterial additives can prevent the microbial metabolism of urinary metabolites, thereby rendering the urine sample suitable for downstream metabolomic applications. In addition, to reduce the metabolite transformation subsequent to sample collection, snap-freezing in liquid nitrogen aids in metabolic quenching (i.e., inactivation of enzymatic reactions), thereby obtaining an accurate picture of the metabolome at sampling time [9, 13].

The health status and fluid intake of sample submitters could also impact the solute concentration of urine. In such situations, pre-analytic normalization is essential to correct for variations in urinary constituents. Urine samples are normalized by measuring the osmolality or specific gravity, and subsequent dilution to the lowest concentration before running samples in separation and detection analytical platforms for metabolomics [9].

4. Analytical techniques used in metabolomics

Metabolomics provides a global analysis of several classes of metabolites with diverse physicochemical characteristics present in any biological sample. In general, metabolomic profiling employs two major analytical techniques for detection of metabolites, such as high-field NMR and MS. Advanced chromatographic separation techniques coupled with the aforesaid spectroscopic or spectrometric methods aid in efficiently separating complex matrices for effective detection. When comparing the detection methods, although NMR is a robust and nondestructive method, it has a lower sensitivity compared to MS. However, NMR is capable of structural elucidation of novel unknown compounds. On the other hand, MS is a very sensitive method that requires sample preparation steps coupled with suitable separation techniques to reduce ion suppression. For untargeted metabolomics, high-resolution MS instrumentation is required, whereas targeted metabolomics employ low-resolution MS platforms [5].

5. Clinical research studies utilizing urine metabolomics as a diagnostic platform

Several research studies have focused on evaluating urinary biomarkers for clinically assessing the progression of a disease or different stages of disease evolution. These biomarkers can aid in the clinical assessment of patients without apparent disease, with suspected disease, or rather the progression or remission of overt disease [14]. The following sections describe some of the clinical conditions that have been studied by researchers for potentially identifying biomarkers in urine for diseases in general, such as cancers, metabolic syndromes, and infectious and renal diseases.

5.1 Cancer

Early advances in metabolomics technology have provided insight into the metabolism of cancer by focusing on how the Warburg effect in cancerous cells uses glycolysis effectively to produce amino acids, nucleotides, and lipids necessary for tumor proliferation. Furthermore, metabolomics research has also been used to discover novel diagnostic cancer biomarkers to better understand its complex heterogeneous nature, to discover pathways involved in cancer that could be used for identification of new targets, and for monitoring metabolic biomarkers for therapeutic aspects of cancer treatment. The metabolomics approach also provides ways to personalized cancer treatments by yielding essential information regarding the cancer patient's response to medical interventions. Urine contains metabolic signatures of many biochemical pathways and thus gives way for a cohesive metabolomic approach. Techniques such as hydrophilic interaction chromatography (HILIC-LC-MS), reversed-phase ultra-performance liquid chromatography (RP-UPLC-MS), and gas chromatography time-of-flight mass spectrometry (GC-TOF-MS) are used for urine analysis [15].

Gas chromatography/mass spectrometry (GC/MS) has been recently used to explore disease biomarkers from urine or serum samples. Both primary and secondary metabolites can be analyzed as a metabolomic approach for biomarker analysis. The importance of early diagnosis is especially true in kidney cancer, especially prior to metastatic spread, and can improve survival rates from 10% to greater than 90%. The ultimate composition of molecules in the urine is the result not only of glomerular filtration but also of tubular secretion and reabsorption. Normal urine contains approximately 150 mg/24 h of protein, and compounds such as inulin (5 kDa) and lysozyme (14 kDa) are reported to appear freely in the urine. Although kidney cancer is the sixth leading cause of cancer death and represents only 3% of cancer incidence, it is a major cause of death in 11,000 patients per year in the United States. The disease is very resistant to chemotherapy, and one-third of the cases are metastatic at diagnosis. Thus when detected with symptoms, prognosis of renal cell carcinoma (RCC) is poor and once metastatic, it has only a 5% five-year survival rate. Therefore, a novel, convenient, and noninvasive approach is essential for identifying RCC at an earlier stage prior to metastasis [16]. Renal cell carcinoma entails abundant primary and secondary metabolites as potential tumor markers. The human kidney injury molecule-1 (hKIM-1), when normalized to creatinine, appears in the urine of RCC patients and disappears or decreases in concentration after nephrectomy. Hence, detection of such metabolites in urine can be crucial to cancer diagnosis. It is highlighted that metabolomics is ideally suited for such approaches and analysis of these small molecule metabolites that appear in both serum and urine can be crucial [15].

Metabolomics has also been used to investigate the urinary metabolite differences between hepatocellular carcinoma (HCC) male patients and normal male subjects. The urinary endogenous metabolome was assayed using chemical derivatization followed by GC/MS. After GC/MS analysis, 103 metabolites were detected, of which 18 metabolites were shown to be significantly different between the HCC and control groups. Subsequently, a diagnostic model was constructed with a combination of 18 marker metabolites. This noninvasive technique of identifying HCC biomarkers from urine has potential application in clinical diagnostic oncology. Overall, these findings underscore that metabolomic analysis is a potent and promising strategy for identifying novel biomarkers of HCC [17].

5.2 Metabolic syndrome

The "metabolic syndrome" (MetS) can be understood as a clustering of components that reflect overnutrition, sedentary lifestyles, and resultant excess adiposity. MetS is a cluster of different conditions and not a single disease. The prevalence of the MetS is increasing to epidemic proportions in the United States and also in developing nations. MetS is associated with doubling of incidence of cardiovascular disease risk and an increased risk for incident type 2 diabetes mellitus [18].

Accurate predictors of cardiometabolic diseases are of particular importance since the condition can be present long before the symptoms become clinically apparent. Nuclear magnetic resonance spectroscopy and gas- or liquid-chromatography coupled with MS are the major platforms applied to identify predictive biomarkers, monitoring therapeutic response as well as in basic mechanism studies of obesity, metabolic syndrome, type 2 diabetes, and cardiometabolic diseases for early diagnosis. Nicotinuric acid is correlated with cardiometabolic risk factors such as body mass index (BMI), blood pressure, HbA1c, blood lipids, and C-reactive protein, thus suggesting that it could be a potential biomarker of important features of MetS such as altered lipid metabolism and increased insulin resistance [18, 19].

Metabolic profiling of urine samples has also been used as a diagnostic tool in the predicting liver disease progression because traditional clinical chemistry tests for liver function only aid in diagnosis after substantial liver damage has occurred. With the current diagnostic methods incapable of predicting typical Jaundice syndrome (JS) in hepatic dysfunction, Wang et al. [20] conducted a study for the identification of potential biomarkers from JS disease by using a nontarget metabolomics method and testing their usefulness in human JS diagnosis. To identify the potential biomarkers, multivariate data analysis methods were utilized revealing 44 marker metabolites contributing to the complete separation of JS from healthy controls [20]. Targeted metabolite analysis revealed alterations in critical JS metabolic pathways, such as glutamate metabolism, synthesis and degradation of ketone bodies, alanine and aspartate metabolism strongly associated with JS development [20]. In another study, researchers compared the urine metabolome panel of three human subject group categories, namely individuals with nonalcoholic fatty liver disease (NAFLD), nonalcoholic steatohepatitis (NASH), as well as age and sex-matched healthy controls. Urine metabolomic analysis performed using tandem LC-MS revealed differences in 31 metabolites between NASH and NAFLD groups, including variations in nucleic acids and amino acids. Among the overlapping metabolites, it was inferred that pathways of energy and amino acid metabolism, as well as the pentose phosphate pathway, were closely associated with progression of NAFLD and NASH [21].

UHPLC-Q-TOF-MS based metabolomics approach was applied to gain understanding of the global profiling of endogenous metabolites in urine from high-fat diet-induced obese rats [22]. Integrated with multivariate analysis, metabolic variations between the obese rats and healthy rats were differentiated. Twenty potential biomarkers were identified in response to high-fat diet-induced obesity. Seventeen of them are novel potential biomarkers that are independent of the known risk indicators for obesity, except hippurate, phenylacetylglutamine (PAG), and creatinine. Using the correlation between these biomarkers, a network diagraph was generated based on search results from the Kyoto Encyclopedia of Genes and Genomes (KEGG) database. Tryptophan metabolism, phenylalanine and tyrosine metabolism, and gut microbiota metabolism were found to be significantly disturbed in obese rats [22].

5.3 Urinary metabolites associated with inflammatory diseases

Immune-mediated inflammatory diseases are a group of diseases that share common molecular mechanisms and are characterized by aberrant and chronic activation of the immune system. Rheumatoid arthritis, psoriasis, psoriatic arthritis, systemic lupus erythematosus, Crohn's disease, and ulcerative colitis are the most prevalent immune-mediated inflammatory diseases. Although these diseases target different tissues and organs, they share many genetic loci, and clinically similar inflammatory diseases are known to share specific hub metabolites such as citrate. Numerous high-throughput analysis technologies are available that can generate comprehensive profiles of multiple metabolites. However, most of these techniques require invasive sampling procedures. Understanding and identifying biological markers in urine that accurately correlate with the inflammatory disease can prove vital for easy and early disease diagnosis under routine clinical settings.

A study conducted by Alonso and coworkers identified multiple urinary metabolites (citrate, alanine, methyl succinate, trigonelline, N-acetyl Amino Acids, and an unknown metabolite) that can be associated with three or more of the immune-mediated inflammatory diseases [23]. Most of these urinary metabolites were found in lower concentrations in patients with inflammatory diseases compared to controls. Citrate, the strongest hub metabolite, for example, was present at lower concentrations in the urine of inflammatory bowel disease, rheumatoid arthritis, and, systemic lupus erythematosus patients [23–25]. Additionally, inflammatory diseases with similar phenotypes exhibited similar urinary metabolomes. Low levels of carnitine were identified in chronic arthritis diseases, namely rheumatoid arthritis and psoriatic arthritis. Similarly, reduced concentrations of hippurate were observed in patients with inflammatory bowel diseases such as Crohn's disease and ulcerative colitis. In short, immune-mediated inflammatory diseases can be aggregated into three distinct clusters based on the urinary metabolite profiles: (1) psoriasis and psoriatic arthritis, (2) Crohn's disease and ulcerative colitis, and (3) rheumatoid arthritis and systemic lupus erythematosus, all sharing between 3 and 6 metabolite associations [23]. However, since the treatment strategies of Crohn's disease and ulcerative colitis are entirely different, a single test that distinguishes the two will be of utmost clinical value. In this context, researchers have identified that hippurate and 4-cresol sulfate levels were lower in patients with Crohn's disease when compared to control and ulcerative colitis patients. Although similar studies showed that urinary metabolome is useful for the differential diagnosis between ulcerative colitis and Crohn's disease, complicated nature of the disease and the confounding factors such as surgical resections, drug and dietary therapy can interfere with the metabolic changes in observational studies. Therefore, the aforesaid confounders should be considered before such analysis [24, 26]. Urinary metabolome also has the potential for predicting both the disease activity and disease recurrence (especially at the site of surgery) in patients with Crohn's disease. For example, metabolites namely citrate, hippurate and 3-hydroxyisovalerate were found in much lower levels in patients with high disease activity for Crohn's disease than in low disease activity for Crohn's disease patients [23, 27]. Higher levels of three urinary metabolites (L-3,4-dihydroxy phenylalanine, levoglucosan, ethyl malonate), and lower concentrations of propylene glycol were associated with endoscopic recurrence in Crohn's s disease in patients who have undergone ileocolonic resection [27]. Furthermore, urinary metabolites, octanoyl glucuronide, pyridoxic acid, and pantothenic acid were shown as dietary biomarkers for clinical remission in pediatric patients with inflammatory bowel disease, who had undergone either exclusive enteral nutrition or corticosteroid therapy [28].

In addition, there are distinct urinary metabolites such as phenyl acetyl glycine and tyrosine that were specific for ulcerative colitis and rheumatoid arthritis, respectively [23]. Urinary excretion of prostaglandins thromboxane synthase and prostacyclin metabolites were increased in patients with severe atherosclerosis [29]. Similarly, elevated levels of acotinic acid, isocitric acid, and citric acid were observed in the urine of osteoarthritic patients and these provide an indication of mitochondrial dysfunction leading to impaired cartilage and chondrocyte metabolism in osteoarthritis. Moreover, significant urinary metabolomic variations in histidine and histamine were observed between two different phenotypes of osteoarthritis (with and without knee effusion) [30]. The NMR-based approach also demonstrated the metabolic fingerprints of urine samples that distinguished chronic inflammatory rheumatoid diseases from healthy individuals. Several urinary metabolites (including leucine, valine, 3-hydroxyisobutyric acid, 3-hydroxyisovaleric acid, glycine, citric acid, creatinine, hippuric acid, and methylnicotinamide) were downregulated in patients with chronic inflammatory rheumatoid diseases. Some of the changes could be explained as a consequence of urinary tract infections, increased demand for muscle turnover events, or due to distal renal tubular acidosis [31]. As for pelvic inflammatory diseases, a clinical trial conducted by Zou and coworkers showed the presence of eighteen differential metabolites in the urine of rats inoculated with *Ureaplasma urealyticum* and pathogenic *Escherichia coli* to mimic multi-pathogenic infection of the upper genital tract leading to pelvic inflammation [32].

5.4 Infectious diseases

Urine metabolomics has been increasingly used for the study of biomarker discovery in infectious diseases, as it offers significant methodological advantages. The application of NMR spectroscopy metabolomics has the potential for infectious disease diagnosis since it can differentiate between various viral and bacterial infections. A specific metabolomic response comes from the host in the form of immune cells and apoptosis signaling when a pathogen causes infection [33, 34].

Urinary tract infection (UTI) is one of the most common bacterial infections in humans. Main causative organisms of UTI include *Escherichia coli, Klebsiella pneumoniae, Pseudomonas aeruginosa, Staphylococcus aureus, and Enterococcus faecalis.* Ultra-Fast Liquid Chromatography Mass Spectrometry (UFLC-MS) was used to differentiate UTI by *E. coli* in a case study involving 17 individuals. Metabolic discriminators identified were related to TCA cycle, terpenoid backbone biosynthesis, amino sugars and nucleotide sugars metabolism, arachidonic acid, and steroid hormone biosynthesis [35]. In another study, nontargeted exploratory UPLC-MS-based approach was used for the investigation of UTI-related changes in urine associated with *E. coli* infection in 117 subjects. A C-terminal glycopeptide of the human fibrinogen alpha-chain was identified as the discriminator metabolite [36]. NMR-based screening showed that *K. pneumoniae* causing UTI can metabolize glycerol to 1,3-propanediol (1,3-PD), acetate, ethanol, and succinate. The quantity of 1,3-PD was found to be proportional to the bacterial count. However, other bacteria causing UTI cannot metabolize glycerol under similar conditions [37, 38]. Urinary NMR spectroscopy of samples infected with *E. coli*, *K. pneumoniae*, *P. aeruginosa*, and *P. mirabilis* showed peaks of nonspecific metabolites such as succinate, acetate, lactate, and ethanol compared to healthy groups in a case-control study done in 617 people. Lactate metabolism, nicotinic acid, and methionine metabolism were altered in the affected individuals [39].

Pneumonia is caused by a wide range of microorganisms, including bacteria, fungi, viruses, and parasites. Conventional methods of diagnosis are time-consuming and include isolation of organisms from blood, sputum, pleural fluid, and bronchoalveolar lavage. Urinary metabolomics can be used as a tool to differentiate *Streptococcus pneumoniae* infection, responsible for community-acquired pneumonia from other infections. A study was conducted on 641 individuals, including healthy volunteers, patients with metabolic stress, fasting individuals, patients with pneumococcal pneumonia, other lung infections, and asthma or chronic obstructive pulmonary disease (COPD). NMR spectra comparison of 61 metabolites in urine from age and gender-matched *S. pneumoniae* infected and noninfected groups were performed. Among these metabolites, 6 were significantly decreased while 27 were significantly increased. Six metabolites that decreased are associated with TCA cycle intermediates (citrate, and succinate), nicotinamide metabolism (1-methylnicotinamide), food intake (levoglucosan and trigonelline), and protein catabolism (1-methylhistidine). Increased concentration was observed in amino acids (alanine, asparagine, isoleucine, leucine, lysine, serine, threonine, tryptophan, tyrosine, and valine), fatty acid oxidation (3-hydroxybutyrate, acetone, carnitine, and acetylcarnitine), inflammation (hypoxanthine and fucose), metabolites involved in glycolysis (glucose and lactate), osmolytes (*myo*-inositol and taurine), acetate, quinolinate, adipate, dimethylamine, and creatine. TCA cycle intermediates 2-oxoglutarate and fumarate also appeared to increase upon pneumococcal infection. Metabolites that were not affected by pneumococcal infection included creatinine, 3-methylhistidine, aconitate (*trans* and *cis*), metabolites related to gut microflora (3-indoxylsulfate, 4-hydroxyphenylacetate, hippurate, formate and TMAO (trimethylamine-*N*-oxide), dietary metabolites (mannitol, propylene glycol, sucrose, and tartrate) and certain amino acids (glycine, glutamine, histidine, and pyroglutamate) [38, 40]. In another study, metabolomic profiling of an independent sample set of 145 urine samples from healthy individuals or patients with various conditions showed around 86% and 94% in sensitivity and specificity, respectively, for the diagnosis of pneumococcal pneumonia [40].

Neonatal sepsis is an infection that occurs in the bloodstream of newborn infants less than 28 days old, and it can be divided into early-onset and late-onset. A case study was conducted to analyze the difference in the urinary metabolome of infected and healthy neonates [41]. Urine metabolic profiles were assessed using nontargeted NMR spectroscopy and targeted liquid chromatography-tandem mass spectrometry analysis in 16 septic neonates and 16 nonseptic ones. The metabolic profile of neonates with sepsis was found to be different compared to those without sepsis. Metabolites from energy-producing biosynthetic pathways and basic structural components of the organism showed clear separation. Elevations in urinary taurine and hypotaurine were noted in septic neonates. Depletion in glutamine levels was also seen in critically ill adults. Hypo- or hyperglycemia was also common in adults. Increased amounts of pyruvate and lactate in the urine can be due to sepsis-associated hypoperfusion and/or hypoxia [42]. In septic preterm infants, early metabolic responses include lactic acidosis and increases glucose requirements. A product of purine degradation called inosine was also observed in higher quantities in this condition because of cellular destruction. Trimethylamine N-oxide (TMAO) levels and certain vitamins such as riboflavin and nicotinamide were found to be reduced in neonatal septic patients [41].

Clostridium difficile is a spore-forming bacterial pathogen, which is the leading cause of healthcare-associated infective diarrhea [43, 44]. In the United States, more than 500,000 cases of *C. difficile* infection (CDI) are reported annually accruing $6.3 billion in healthcare costs [44]. Intestinal dysbiosis is the reason for recurrent CDI. Urinary metabolites might be used as a prognostic method for patients with recurrent CDI as no diagnostic tests are available to predict the risk of CDI recurrences in patients [45]. With regards to *C. difficile* infections, Kao *et al.* performed NMR studies on urine of 31 infected subjects (age- and sex-matched to 31 healthy controls) and detected 53 metabolites. Choline appeared to be the most relevant for the diagnosis of *C. difficile* infection. This finding has been possibly attributed to the absence of choline-metabolizing microorganisms in this infection [33]. Isa *et al.* proposed four urinary metabolites as biomarkers for active tuberculosis patients [46]. Using an untargeted HPLC-MS and MS/MS, 102 urine samples were collected from infected individuals. The majority of the metabolites were neopterin, kynurenine, spermine, *N*-acetylated sugars, and sialic acids, which are host-derived metabolites involved in immune cell activation [46].

COVID 19 is a pneumonia caused by coronavirus (SARS-CoV 2) responsible for producing a global pandemic and still continues to be a worldwide emergency [47]. During SARS-CoV-2 infection, research studies have been conducted to correlate urinary constituent abnormalities for COVID 19 disease severity and outcome. A case study was done in four cohorts namely, healthy control (n = 27), non-COVID-19 control (n = 17), patients with nonsevere COVID-19 (n = 48), and patients with severe COVID-19 (n = 23) [48]. Peptide yields from urine samples in patients with severe and nonsevere cases were found to be greater compared to serum samples in the healthy control group. A total of 16,148 peptides and 1494 proteins were obtained from sera using tandem mass-tag (TMT)-based proteomics, while 19,732 peptides and 3854 proteins were identified from urine. Similarly, 80% of detectable serum proteins and 62% of serum metabolites were found in urine of the infected group. Cytoplasmic proteins (26%) and membrane proteins (21%) were the most abundant protein groups in the urinary proteome, whereas the proportion of secreted proteins was only 16%. Further, more intracellular compartment proteins released from tissues were seen in the urinary proteome of the infected group compared to the serum proteome. Also, 197 cytokines and their receptors were observed in urine of infected group, whereas 124 cytokines were seen in serum. In the same study, the reduction in endosomal sorting complexes required for transport (ESCRT) complex proteins and downregulation of CXCL14 in urine was reported to be associated with an increase in SARS-CoV-2 replication [48]. In another study consisting of 142 infected volunteers and 104 healthy volunteers, urine samples were subjected to mass spectrometry. Significant alterations in nitrogen metabolism, D-glutamine and D-glutamate metabolism, aminoacyl-tRNA biosynthesis, arginine biosynthesis, glutathione metabolism, pantothenate and CoA biosynthesis, glyoxylate and dicarboxylate metabolism were noticed among infected group and control group. Nineteen amino acids such as alanine, leucine, glutamine, tryptophan, and 15 acylcarnitines were obtained from urine analysis. Glycine level was decreased in the infected group. Alteration in valine was also observed. This study suggested acylcarnitines as important markers for COVID-19 infection [49].

Acquired Immunodeficiency Syndrome (AIDS) is responsible for causing a severe immunosuppressive state on the immune system of humans. AIDS has emerged as a global health hazard and no effective methods are available for the characterization of affected patients. Urinary metabolomics can be a promising method to differentiate affected and nonaffected AIDS individuals, and also for monitoring the progress of HIV therapeutics. Studies using biofluids, such as urine, whole blood, and serum, have also been employed to identify metabolite markers correlating to HIV-induced oxidative stress (OS). Munshi et al. suggested that urinary neopterin could be used as a metabolic biomarker of AIDS infection. Urinary glutamic acid and formic acid levels were higher in HIV/AIDS patients compared to healthy controls. When comparing HIV-infected patients treated with or without antiretroviral therapy (ART), ART naïve patients had lower levels of urinary methionine, 2-methylglutaric acid, L-alanine, and glycolic acid, however, patients receiving ART had even reduced levels of the aforesaid metabolites [50]. Hence, urinary amino acids and their metabolites can help to serve as markers for assessing the progress of ART in AIDS patients.

Malaria is a mosquito-borne parasitic illness caused by *Plasmodium falciparum*, *Plasmodium vivax*, and *Plasmodium berghei*. Morbidity and mortality caused by these parasites are greater in tropical and sub-tropical countries. Prospect of infection biomarkers in biofluids is therefore important in a population to control the impact of the infection. Urinary metabolites could be used as a tool to differentiate the infected groups from the noninfected ones. In a case-control study of 21 *P. falciparum*-infected individuals and 25 controls, urine samples subjected to high-performance liquid chromatography-high resolution mass spectrometry (HPLC/HRMS) revealed altered levels of 1,3-diacetylpropane, *N*-acetylputrescine, and *N*-acetylspermidine between patients and control cohorts, thereby suggesting these molecules as potential biomarkers for malarial infections [51]. NMR spectroscopy of urinary samples from patients infected with *P. vivax* was also studied. Urinary ornithine and pipecolic acid were higher in malarial patients and could be used as a potential biomarker to differentiate between malarial and nonmalarial cases [52]. In another study using a mouse model of *P. berghei* infection, 4-amino-1-[3-hydroxy-5-(hydroxymethyl)-2,3-dihydrofuran-2-yl]pyrimidin-2(1H)-one and 2-amino-4-({[5-(4-amino-2-oxopyrimidin-1(2H)-yl)-4-hydroxy-4,5-dihydrofuran-2-yl]methyl}sulfanyl) butanoic acid were the two urinary metabolites detected in infected mice groups compared to healthy mice [53]. Therefore, the aforementioned catabolites in urine may aid to assess the progression of the disease among affected individuals.

5.5 Renal dysfunction

Acute kidney injury is defined as a sudden phase of kidney failure that occurs in a few hours. This condition is characterized by an increase in serum creatinine and a notable decrease in urine output [54]. Chronic kidney disease (CKD) is a condition, where glomerular filtration rate is progressively affected along with kidney damage [55]. In a study conducted in patients with acute kidney injury, urine samples from patients subjected to LC-MS and 1H NMR scanning revealed an increase in urea cycle, proline metabolism, nitric oxide pathway, and its metabolite, asymmetric dimethyl-arginine (ADMA), serotonin metabolism and homovanillic acid. On the other hand, a decrease in Kreb's cycle and citrate, benzoate metabolism and hippurate, pyruvate metabolism, and lactate were observed [56–58]. In another study conducted by Matin-Lorenzo et al., urine samples were collected from 24 control subjects and 38 patients with acute kidney injury. LC-MS/MS analysis revealed urinary 2-hydroxybutyric acid, pantothenic acid, and hippuric acid were significantly downregulated and urinary N-acetylneuraminic acid, phosphoethanolamine and serine were upregulated in diseased patients [59]. It was also reported that a low risk of chronic kidney disease is associated with urinary glycine and histidine, increased urinary lysine, and NG-monomethyl-L-arginine (NMMA) [60]. However, carnitine metabolism, beta-oxidation and acylcarnitines, phenylacetylglutamine, urea cycle, proline metabolism and their metabolites, proline, and citrulline were increased in chronic kidney disease. Conversely, urea cycle, proline metabolism, nitric oxide pathway and ADMA, Krebs cycle and citrate, bile acid metabolism, and taurocholate were reported down-regulated in chronic kidney disease conditions [61, 62].

Diabetes is a chronic (DM) metabolic disease that result in unusually higher preprandial plasma glucose levels as a result of defects in insulin secretion, insulin activity, or both. Chronic diabetes can lead to several pathophysiological conditions that range from cardiovascular abnormalities to renal failure. The hemodynamic dysregulation caused by diabetes mediates renal injury by inducing abnormal morphological and functional changes in the renal nephrons [63]. Gas chromatography-mass spectrometry was used to quantify 94 urine metabolites in screening cohorts of patients with diabetes mellitus (DM) and chronic kidney disease CKD (DM + CKD), in patients with DM without CKD (DM–CKD), and in healthy controls. Thirteen metabolites were significantly reduced in the DM + CKD cohorts compared to healthy groups. Twelve of them are related to mitochondrial metabolism, suggesting a suppression of mitochondrial activity in diabetic kidney disease [64].

Autosomal dominant polycystic disease is a hereditary disorder which is characterized by cyst formation in ductal organs, mainly the kidney and the liver, and also by gastrointestinal, musculoskeletal, and cardiovascular abnormalities [65], Research conducted in a mouse model for autosomal dominant polycystic kidney disease was used to assess whether metabolomic shifts prior to renal cystogenesis can aid in early diagnosis for the condition. Utilizing GC-MS time of flight spectroscopy, urine samples collected from mice prior to exhibiting any serological evidence of kidney dysfunction revealed that purine and galactose metabolic pathways were affected, with elevation of biomarkers such as allantoic and adenosine [66].

6. Conclusion

Urine metabolomics is a powerful diagnostic technique that can be utilized to diagnose several diseases, including cancers, hereditary diseases, immune-mediated and metabolic disorders, and renal dysfunction. Urine metabolite constituents essentially serve as biomarker signatures to identify pathways related to specific diseases as well as to detect abnormal concentrations of the metabolites that may be associated with the disease. Furthermore, the analysis of urinary metabolome can be used to evaluate disease activity, response to treatments and to monitor the progression or remission of the disease. Additionally, the standardization and curation of urine metabolomic databases for health and pathological phenotypes can potentially be developed and employed in routine clinical settings for disease diagnosis.

Conflict of interest

The authors declare no conflict of interest.

Author details

Abraham Joseph Pellissery[1], Poonam Gopika Vinayamohan[2], Leya Susan Viju[3], Divya Joseph[3] and Kumar Venkitanarayanan[3]*

1 Department of Comparative, Diagnostic and Population Medicine, College of Veterinary Medicine, University of Florida, Gainesville, FL, USA

2 Department of Preventive Medicine, College of Veterinary Medicine, Ohio State University, Colombus, OH, USA

3 Department of Animal Science, University of Connecticut. Storrs, CT, USA

*Address all correspondence to: kumar.venkitanarayanan@uconn.edu

References

[1] Haber MH. Pisse prophecy: A brief history of urinalysis. Clinics in Laboratory Medicine. 1988;**8**:415-430

[2] Bolodeoku J, Donaldson D. Urinalysis in clinical diagnosis. Journal of Clinical Pathology. 1996;**49**:623-626

[3] Echeverry G, Hortin GL, Rai AJ. Introduction to urinalysis: Historical perspectives and clinical application. Methods in Molecular Biology. 2010;**641**:1-12. DOI: 10.1007/978-1-60761-711-2_1

[4] Bouatra S, Aziat F, Mandal R, Guo AC, Wilson MR, Knox C, et al. The human urine metabolome. PLoS One. 2013;**8**. DOI: 10.1371/journal.pone.0073076

[5] Segers K, Declerck S, Mangelings D, Heyden YV, Eeckhaut AV. Analytical techniques for metabolomic studies: A review. Bioanalysis. 2019;**11**:2297-2318. DOI: 10.4155/bio-2019-0014

[6] Thévenot EA, Roux A, Xu Y, Ezan E, Junot C. Analysis of the human adult urinary metabolome variations with age, body mass index, and gender by implementing a comprehensive workflow for univariate and OPLS statistical analyses. Journal of Proteome Research. 2015;**14**:3322-3335. DOI: 10.1021/acs.jproteome.5b00354

[7] Ryan D, Robards K, Prenzler PD, Kendall M. Recent and potential developments in the analysis of urine: A review. Analytica Chimica Acta. 2011;**684**:17-29. DOI: 10.1016/j.aca.2010.10.035

[8] Zhang A, Sun H, Wu X, Wang X. Urine metabolomics. Clinica Chimica Acta. 2012;**414**:65-69. DOI: 10.1016/J.CCA.2012.08.016

[9] Chetwynd AJ, Dunn WB, Rodriguez-Blanco G. Collection and preparation of clinical samples for metabolomics. In: Advances in Experimental Medicine and Biology. Vol. 965. Springer New York LLC; 2017. pp. 19-44. DOI: 10.1007/978-3-319-47656-8_2

[10] Idle JR, Gonzalez FJ. Metabolomics. Cell Metabolism. 2007;**6**:348-351. DOI: 10.1016/j.cmet.2007.10.005

[11] Lichtenberg S, Trifonova OP, Maslov DL, Balashova EE, Lokhov PG. Metabolomic laboratory-developed tests: Current status and perspectives. Metabolites. 2021;**11**:423. DOI: 10.3390/metabo11070423

[12] Ren S, Hinzman AA, Kang EL, Szczesniak RD, Lu LJ. Computational and statistical analysis of metabolomics data. Metabolomics. 2015;**11**:1492-1513. DOI: 10.1007/s11306-015-0823-6

[13] González-Domínguez R, González-Domínguez Á, Sayago A, Fernández-Recamales Á. Recommendations and best practices for standardizing the pre-analytical processing of blood and urine samples in metabolomics. Metabolites. 2020;**10**:1-18. DOI: 10.3390/metabo10060229

[14] Roberts LD, Gerszten RE. Toward new biomarkers of cardiometabolic diseases. Cell Metabolism. 2013;**18**:43-50. DOI: 10.1016/j.cmet.2013.05.009

[15] Kind T, Tolstikov V, Fiehn O, Weiss RH. A comprehensive urinary metabolomic approach for identifying kidney cancer. Analytical Biochemistry. 2007;**363**:185-195. DOI: 10.1016/j.ab.2007.01.028

[16] Kim K, Aronov P, Zakharkin SO, Anderson D, Perroud B, Thompson IM, et al. Urine metabolomics analysis for kidney cancer detection and biomarker discovery. Molecular and Cellular Proteomics. 2009;**8**:558-570. DOI: 10.1074/mcp.M800165-MCP200

[17] Wang X, Zhang A, Sun H. Power of metabolomics in diagnosis and biomarker discovery of hepatocellular carcinoma. Hepatology. 2013;**57**:2072-2077. DOI: 10.1002/hep.26130

[18] Cornier MA, Dabelea D, Hernandez TL, Lindstrom RC, Steig AJ, Stob NR, et al. The metabolic syndrome. Endocrine Reviews. 2008;**29**:777-822. DOI: 10.1210/er.2008-0024

[19] Wu Q, Li J, Sun X, He D, Cheng Z, Li J, et al. Multi-stage metabolomics and genetic analyses identified metabolite biomarkers of metabolic syndrome and their genetic determinants. eBioMedicine. 2021;**74**. DOI: 10.1016/j.ebiom.2021.103707

[20] Wang X, Zhang A, Han Y, Wang P, Sun H, Song G, et al. Urine metabolomics analysis for biomarker discovery and detection of jaundice syndrome in patients with liver disease. Molecular and Cellular Proteomics. 2012;**11**:370-380. DOI: 10.1074/mcp.M111.016006

[21] Dong S, Zhan ZY, Cao HY, Wu C, Bian YQ, Li JY, et al. Urinary metabolomics analysis identifies key biomarkers of different stages of nonalcoholic fatty liver disease. World Journal of Gastroenterology. 2017;**23**:2771-2784. DOI: 10.3748/wjg.v23.i15.2771

[22] Men L, Pi Z, Zhou Y, Wei M, Liu Y, Song F, et al. Urine metabolomics of high-fat diet induced obesity using UHPLC-Q-TOF-MS. Journal of Pharmaceutical and Biomedical Analysis. 2017;**132**:258-266. DOI: 10.1016/j.jpba.2016.10.012

[23] Alonso A, Julià A, Vinaixa M, Domènech E, Fernández-Nebro A, Cañete JD, et al. Urine metabolome profiling of immune-mediated inflammatory diseases. BMC Medicine. 2016;**14**:133. DOI: 10.1186/s12916-016-0681-8

[24] Stephens NS, Siffledeen J, Su X, Murdoch TB, Fedorak RN, Slupsky CM. Urinary NMR metabolomic profiles discriminate inflammatory bowel disease from healthy. Journal of Crohn's and Colitis. 2013;7. DOI: 10.1016/j.crohns.2012.04.019

[25] Dawiskiba T, Deja S, Mulak A, Zabek A, Jawień E, Pawełka D, et al. Serum and urine metabolomic fingerprinting in diagnostics of inflammatory bowel diseases. World Journal of Gastroenterology. 2014;**20**:163-174. DOI: 10.3748/wjg.v20.i1.163

[26] Williams HR, Cox JI, Walker DG, North BV, Patel VM, Marshall SE, et al. Characterization of inflammatory bowel disease with urinary metabolic profiling. Official Journal of the American College of Gastroenterology|ACG. 2009;**104**:1435-1444

[27] Keshteli AH, Tso R, Dieleman LA, Park H, Kroeker KI, Jovel J, et al. A distinctive urinary metabolomic fingerprint is linked with endoscopic postoperative disease recurrence in Crohn's disease patients. Inflammatory Bowel Diseases. 2018;**24**:861-870. DOI: 10.1093/ibd/izx070

[28] Yamamoto M, Shanmuganathan M, Hart L, Pai N, Britz-McKibbin P. Urinary metabolites enable differential diagnosis and therapeutic monitoring of Pediatric inflammatory bowel disease.

Metabolites. 2021;**11**:245. DOI: 10.3390/metabo11040245

[29] Reilly IA, Doran JB, Smith B, FitzGerald GA. Increased thromboxane biosynthesis in a human preparation of platelet activation: Biochemical and functional consequences of selective inhibition of thromboxane synthase. Circulation. 1986;**73**:1300-1309. DOI: 10.1161/01.cir.73.6.1300

[30] Li X, Yang S, Qiu Y, Zhao T, Chen T, Su M, et al. Urinary metabolomics as a potentially novel diagnostic and stratification tool for knee osteoarthritis. Metabolomics. 2010;**6**:109-118. DOI: 10.1007/s11306-009-0184-0

[31] Vignoli A, Rodio DM, Bellizzi A, Sobolev AP, Anzivino E, Mischitelli M, et al. NMR-based metabolomic approach to study urine samples of chronic inflammatory rheumatic disease patients. Analytical and Bioanalytical Chemistry. 2017;**409**:1405-1413. DOI: 10.1007/s00216-016-0074-z

[32] Zou W, Wen X, Sheng X, Zheng Y, Xiao Z, Luo J, et al. Gas chromatography-mass spectrometric method-based urine metabolomic profile of rats with pelvic inflammatory disease. Experimental and Therapeutic Medicine. 2016;**11**:1653-1660. DOI: 10.3892/etm.2016.3112

[33] Tounta V, Liu Y, Cheyne A, Larrouy-Maumus G. Metabolomics in infectious diseases and drug discovery. Molecular Omics. 2021;**17**:376-393. DOI: 10.1039/d1mo00017a

[34] Gupta A, Bansal N, Houston B. Metabolomics of urinary tract infection: A new uroscope in town. Expert Review of Molecular Diagnostics. 2012;**12**:361-370. DOI: 10.1586/erm.12.27

[35] Lv H, Hung CS, Chaturvedi KS, Hooton TM, Henderson JP. Development of an integrated metabolomic profiling approach for infectious diseases research. Analyst. 2011;**136**:4752-4763. DOI: 10.1039/c1an15590c

[36] Pacchiarotta T, Hensbergen PJ, Wuhrer M, Van Nieuwkoop C, Nevedomskaya E, Derks RJE, et al. Fibrinogen alpha chain O-glycopeptides as possible markers of urinary tract infection. Journal of Proteomics. 2012;**75**:1067-1073. DOI: 10.1016/j.jprot.2011.10.021

[37] Gupta A, Dwivedi M, Gowda GAN, Mahdi AA, Jain A, Ayyagari A, et al. 1H NMR spectroscopy in the diagnosis of Klebsiella pneumoniae-induced urinary tract infection. NMR in Biomedicine. 2006;**19**:1055-1061. DOI: 10.1002/nbm.1078

[38] Pacchiarotta T, Deelder AM, Mayboroda OA. Metabolomic investigations of human infections. Bioanalysis. 2012;**4**:919-925. DOI: 10.4155/bio.12.61

[39] Gupta A, Dwivedi M, Mahdi AA, Gowda GAN, Khetrapal CL, Bhandari M. 1H-nuclear magnetic resonance spectroscopy for identifying and quantifying common uropathogens: A metabolic approach to the urinary tract infection. BJU International. 2009;**104**:236-244. DOI: 10.1111/j.1464-410X.2009.08448.x

[40] Slupsky CM, Rankin KN, Fu H, Chang D, Rowe BH, Charles PGP, et al. Pneumococcal pneumonia: Potential for diagnosis through a urinary metabolic profile. Journal of Proteome Research. 2009;**8**:5550-5558. DOI: 10.1021/pr9006427

[41] Sarafidis K, Chatziioannou AC, Thomaidou A, Gika H, Mikros E, Benaki D, et al. Urine metabolomics in neonates with late-onset sepsis in a

case-control study. Scientific Reports. 2017;7. DOI: 10.1038/srep45506

[42] Su L, Li H, Xie A, Liu D, Rao W, Lan L, et al. Dynamic changes in amino acid concentration profiles in patients with sepsis. PLoS One. 2015;**10**. DOI: 10.1371/journal.pone.0121933

[43] Smits WK, Lyras D, Lacy DB, Wilcox MH, Kuijper EJ. Clostridium difficile infection. Nature Reviews Disease Primers. 2016;**2**:1-20. DOI: 10.1038/nrdp.2016.20

[44] Pellissery AJ, Vinayamohan PG, Yin HB, Mooyottu S, Venkitanarayanan K. In vitro efficacy of sodium selenite in reducing toxin production, spore outgrowth and antibiotic resistance in hypervirulent clostridium difficile. Journal of Medical Microbiology. 2019;**68**:1118-1128. DOI: 10.1099/jmm.0.001008

[45] Kao D, Ismond KP, Tso V, Millan B, Hotte N, Fedorak RN. Urine-based metabolomic analysis of patients with Clostridium difficile infection: A pilot study. Metabolomics. 2016;**12**. DOI: 10.1007/s11306-016-1080-z

[46] Isa F, Collins S, Lee MH, Decome D, Dorvil N, Joseph P, et al. Mass spectrometric identification of urinary biomarkers of pulmonary tuberculosis. eBioMedicine. 2018;**31**:157-165. DOI: 10.1016/j.ebiom.2018.04.014

[47] Yang L, Liu S, Liu J, Zhang Z, Wan X, Huang B, et al. COVID-19: Immunopathogenesis and Immunotherapeutics. Signal transduction and targeted. Therapy. 2020;**5**. DOI: 10.1038/s41392-020-00243-2

[48] Bi X, Liu W, Ding X, Liang S, Zheng Y, Zhu X, et al. Proteomic and metabolomic profiling of urine uncovers immune responses in patients with COVID-19. Cell Reports. 2022;**38**. DOI: 10.1016/j.celrep.2021.110271

[49] Barberis E, Timo S, Amede E, Vanella VV, Puricelli C, Cappellano G, et al. Large-scale plasma analysis revealed new mechanisms and molecules associated with the host response to SARS-CoV-2. International Journal of Molecular Sciences. 2020;**21**:8623. DOI: 10.3390/ijms21228623

[50] Munshi SU, Rewari BB, Bhavesh NS, Jameel S. Nuclear magnetic resonance based profiling of biofluids reveals metabolic dysregulation in HIV-infected persons and those on anti-retroviral therapy. PLoS One. 2013;**8**. DOI: 10.1371/journal.pone.0064298

[51] Abdelrazig S, Ortori CA, Davey G, Deressa W, Mulleta D, Barrett DA, et al. A metabolomic analytical approach permits identification of urinary biomarkers for *Plasmodium falciparum* infection: A case-control study. Malaria Journal. 2017;**16**:1-8. DOI: 10.1186/s12936-017-1875-z

[52] Sengupta A, Ghosh S, Basant A, Malusare S, Johri P, Pathak S, et al. Global host metabolic response to *Plasmodium vivax* infection: A 1H NMR based urinary metabonomic study. Malaria Journal. 2011;**10**. DOI: 10.1186/1475-2875-10-384

[53] Tritten L, Keiser J, Godejohann M, Utzinger J, Vargas M, Beckonert O, et al. Metabolic profiling framework for discovery of candidate diagnostic markers of malaria. Scientific Reports. 2013;**3**. DOI: 10.1038/srep02769

[54] Chawla LS, Eggers PW, Star RA, Kimmel PL. Acute kidney injury and chronic kidney disease as interconnected syndromes. New England Journal of Medicine. 2014;**371**:58-66. DOI: 10.1056/nejmra1214243

[55] Webster AC, Nagler EV, Morton RL, Masson P. Chronic kidney disease. Lancet. 2017;**389**:1238-1252. DOI: 10.1016/S0140-6736(16)32064-5

[56] Barrios C, Spector TD, Menni C. Blood, urine and faecal metabolite profiles in the study of adult renal disease. Archives of Biochemistry and Biophysics. 2016;**589**:81-92. DOI: 10.1016/j.abb.2015.10.006

[57] Klawitter J, Haschke M, Kahle C, Dingmann C, Klawitter J, Leibfritz D, et al. Toxicodynamic effects of ciclosporin are reflected by metabolite profiles in the urine of healthy individuals after a single dose. British Journal of Clinical Pharmacology. 2010;**70**:241-251. DOI: 10.1111/j. 1365-2125.2010.03689.x

[58] Bairaktari E, Seferiadis K, Liamis G, Psihogios N, Tsolas O, Elisaf M. Rhabdomyolysis-related renal tubular damage studied by proton nuclear magnetic resonance spectroscopy of urine. Clinical Chemistry. 2002;**48**:1106-1109

[59] Martin-Lorenzo M, Gonzalez-Calero L, Ramos-Barron A, Sanchez-Niño MD, Gomez-Alamillo C, García-Segura JM, et al. Urine metabolomics insight into acute kidney injury point to oxidative stress disruptions in energy generation and H2S availability. Journal of Molecular Medicine. 2017;**95**:1399-1409. DOI: 10.1007/s00109-017-1594-5

[60] McMahon GM, Hwang SJ, Clish CB, Tin A, Yang Q, Larson MG, et al. Urinary metabolites along with common and rare genetic variations are associated with incident chronic kidney disease. Kidney International. 2017;**91**:1426-1435. DOI: 10.1016/j.kint.2017.01.007

[61] Duranton F, Lundin U, Gayrard N, Mischak H, Aparicio M, Mourad G, et al. Plasma and urinary amino acid metabolomic profiling in patients with different levels of kidney function. Clinical Journal of the American Society of Nephrology. 2014;**9**:37-45. DOI: 10.2215/CJN.06000613

[62] Nkuipou-Kenfack E, Duranton F, Gayrard N, Argilés À, Lundin U, Weinberger KM, et al. Assessment of metabolomic and proteomic biomarkers in detection and prognosis of progression of renal function in chronic kidney disease. PLoS One. 2014;**9**. DOI: 10.1371/journal.pone.0096955

[63] Fakhruddin S, Alanazi W, Jackson KE. Diabetes-induced reactive oxygen species: Mechanism of their generation and role in renal injury. Journal Diabetes Research. 2017;**2017**:8379327. DOI: 10.1155/2017/8379327

[64] Sharma K, Karl B, Mathew AV, Gangoiti JA, Wassel CL, Saito R, et al. Metabolomics reveals signature of mitochondrial dysfunction in diabetic kidney disease. Journal of the American Society of Nephrology. 2013;**24**:1901-1912. DOI: 10.1681/ASN.2013020126

[65] Gabow PA. Polycystic kidney disease: Clues to pathogenesis. Kidney International. 1991;**40**:989-996. DOI: 10.1038/ki.1991.306

[66] Taylor SL, Ganti S, Bukanov NO, Chapman A, Fiehn O, Osier M, et al. A metabolomics approach using juvenile cystic mice to identify urinary biomarkers and altered pathways in polycystic kidney disease. American Journal of Physiology. Renal Physiology. 2010;**298**:909-922. DOI: 10.1152/ajprenal.00722.2009.-Autosomal

Chapter 6

Detecting Naloxone in Adulterated Urine Samples: Can Naloxone Be Detected When Buprenorphine/Naloxone Film Is Dipped Directly into Urine and Water?

Hiroko Furo, Tony Lin, Yi Yuan Zhou and Sarah Abdelsayed

Abstract

This study is aimed at exploring if "naloxone" is detected in urine and water samples by dipping buprenorphine/naloxone film directly into these specimens. This study utilized 12 urine samples from 12 healthy participants who were not taking any medications with four samples added as a control. Sublingual generic buprenorphine/naloxone (8 mg/2 mg) film was dipped directly into these samples. They were sent to the ARUP laboratory for gas chromatography-mass spectrometry (GC/MS) quantitative analysis. The results were analyzed using IBM SPSS Statistics software. The results showed that "naloxone" was detected at high levels both in urine samples and in water, into which buprenorphine/naloxone film was dipped. In addition, the "naloxone" level was associated with the area of the film and the time in contact with the urine or water samples, but it was not affected by the urine concentration or the temperature of the specimens. This information will be useful for clinicians in identifying urine manipulation and interpreting urine drug test results and can help them for accurate monitoring of their patients' treatment progress in opioid use disorder (OUD) treatment programs.

Keywords: opioid, urine, buprenorphine, norbuprenorphine, creatinine

1. Introduction

Naloxone* is an opioid antagonist that binds to *mu*-opioid receptors and blocks opioid agonist effect. It is primarily metabolized by the liver and excreted by the kidneys. In the liver, it predominantly undergoes glucuronide conjugation to "naloxone-β-3-glucuronide", while minor metabolic pathways generate nornaloxone

* In order to differentiate "naloxone" found in urine versus other naloxone format such as naloxone in buprenorphine/naloxone combined medication, "naloxone" and other components found in specimens are expressed with quotation marks around them as "naloxone."

(noroxymorphone) through N-dealkylation of naloxone by CYP2C18 and 2C19 primarily, which go through subsequent glucuronidation [1, 2].

Naloxone has approximately 30–45 minute duration of action with a short half-life of 1.87–5.45 hours and reaches peak activity within 0.750–1.13 hours when taken sublingually [2–4]. It dissociates rapidly from opioid receptors within 6.5 minutes and has a low bioavailability of an estimated 3% through the sublingual route of administration with extensive first-pass metabolism [5]. Naloxone can be administered through various routes, which include intravenous, intramuscular, subcutaneous, endotracheal, sublingual, intralingual, submental and intranasal routes [6]. Naloxone, however, is estimated to be 50–250 times more potent when intravenously injected than orally administered [7]. Given this unique characteristic, naloxone is administered parenterally in order to increase its bioavailability, especially when it is used to reverse opioid effect in opioid overdose cases [8].

The effect of naloxone in combined buprenorphine/naloxone medication when taken sublingually is assumed to be clinically insignificant due to its poor absorption (<10%) and extensive first pass metabolism [4]. Therefore, combining buprenorphine and naloxone is strategized to deter unintended use such as intravenous injection and intranasal insufflation [9]. When taken through these routes, the addition of naloxone to buprenorphine antagonizes *mu*-opioid receptors and prevent the intoxicating effects of buprenorphine; however, there are some controversies in adding naloxone to buprenorphine products [5, 10].

While it is widely accepted that naloxone has a poor oral and sublingual bioavailability, many studies found "naloxone" detected at various levels in urine samples of patients who are on sublingual buprenorphine/naloxone medication [11, 12]. For example, Strickland and Burson found that 92.7% of urine samples from those who were on buprenorphine/naloxone medication had >30 ng/mL of "naloxone" detected [13]. At high levels within the system, naloxone may exert its antagonist effect on *mu*-opioid receptors, competing with the desired therapeutic effect of buprenorphine [7]. Therefore, it has been argued that combined medications can still contribute to certain negative effects of naloxone such as precipitated withdrawal during buprenorphine/naloxone induction or maintenance phase of OUD treatment [14].

In addition, many means of urine adulteration among the OUD patients who are on buprenorphine have been reported. One of the common methods of urine adulteration is "dipping" or "spiking" in which patients attempt to dissolve buprenorphine/naloxone film into urine samples directly. Heikman et al. reported that stable patients who are on buprenorphine/naloxone treatment had a median urine "naloxone" concentration of 60 ng/mL while that of unstable patients had a similar median of 70 ng/mL. The same study also found that the urine "naloxone" concentration in unstable patients ranged between 10 and 1700 ng/mL while that of the stable patients had a narrower window between 5 and 200 ng/mL [15]. This contrasting comparison of urine "naloxone" concentrations between stable and unstable patients raises the question of appropriate use of buprenorphine/naloxone therapy and the possibility of high "naloxone" levels in urine as an indication for urine adulteration.

Urine testing strategies have been developed to address this practice. Many previous studies discussed the use of elevated ratio between "buprenorphine" and "norbuprenorphine" in the urine as an indicator of urine adulteration [16–19]. In addition to this high ratio between "buprenorphine" to "norbuprenorphine", high "naloxone" levels in urine samples may also point to adulteration. Warrington, et al. suggested that urine samples with "naloxone" concentration greater than 2000 ng/mL should raise suspicion of adulteration, likely from dipping buprenorphine/naloxone film into the sample [20]. In their study, "buprenorphine" to "norbuprenorphine" ratios were found to be high along with the elevated "naloxone" levels in the urine samples with suspected adulteration. This supports the notion that "naloxone" concentration in the urine can be used as one of the indicators for urine sample adulteration.

While previous studies utilized urine samples from individuals who were on prescribed buprenorphine/naloxone, the impact of adulteration on substance-free urine and purified water remains unproven. Burns et al. conducted an in vitro study in which naloxone was added to urine samples that came from healthy volunteers who were not on any medications, and they found that "naloxone" was detected in the urine samples [21]. While the elevated "naloxone" level in urine samples may be flagged for adulteration, to our knowledge, there are no studies to date that demonstrate whether high levels of "naloxone" can be detected by dipping buprenorphine/naloxone film in water or urine samples from those who are not taking the combination medication.

The aim of this study is to detect and quantify the presence of "naloxone" in adulterated urine samples from those who are not on buprenorphine/naloxone medication and adulterated purified water samples. The findings of this study should deepen our understanding on the pharmacokinetics and pharmacodynamics of naloxone.

2. Methods

2.1 Data

This is a urine test experiment study. After the Institutional Review Board (IRB) application was approved at the University of Texas Health at San Antonio (IRB Protocol ID 20220593HU), 12 urine samples from 12 participants were collected at our clinic. These participants were recruited through flyers and word-of-mouth. One of the inclusion criteria stipulates that the participant is not taking any medications or illegal substances such as opioids and marijuana. This criterion was included because certain medications and substances can inhibit or induce relevant CYP450, which might affect naloxone metabolism and consequently the "naloxone" levels in urine [12]. Another inclusion criterion was "healthy" participants without any major health issues. This inclusion criterion was added because naloxone is metabolized in the liver through glucuronide conjugation, and hepatic impairment can alter naloxone metabolism and consequently affect "naloxone" levels in the urine [22]. The last inclusion criterion was the ability to provide >80 mL urine samples. 15 healthy participants who were not on any medications were initially recruited. 3 participants from this initial pool were excluded due to their inability to provide adequate urine volume. Therefore, 12 urine samples from 12 participants were included in this study. At the time of urine collection, these 12 participants were asked to fill out a demographic information form. Their participation to this study was compensated financially for their time and urine sample contribution.

After the 12-urine samples were collected, each sample was then divided into four specimen aliquots with 20 mL each. Then, sublingual generic buprenorphine/naloxone (8 mg/2 mg) film of 12.8 mm width and 22.0 mm length was dipped directly into each urine specimen. In the first aliquot, 1 mm of buprenorphine/naloxone film was vertically dipped into the urine specimen for three seconds (1 mm*3 sec); in the second, half of a film, approximately 11 mm, was vertically dipped for three seconds (half*3 sec); in the third, a full film was dipped for three seconds (full*3 sec); and in the fourth, a full film was dipped for thirty seconds (full*30 sec). That way, we could investigate if area and/or duration of dipping can alter the "naloxone" levels. In addition, four control samples were utilized; (1) room temperature purified water (RT water), (2) water at approximately 97° F (Body Temperature or BT water), (3) 2 mL of urine diluted with 18 mL RT water (10% RT), and (4) 2 mL of urine diluted with BT 18 mL water (10% BT). These four control samples were added to examine if "naloxone" can be detected in water without any human urine and if the temperature and concentration of urine can affect "naloxone" levels in adulterated urine samples.

2.2 Data analysis

All specimens mentioned above were sent to the ARUP laboratory for quantitative tests. The tests included "naloxone" and "creatinine" levels. The results were stored in **Microsoft Excel (Microsoft 365)** without any identification of the participants. Then, the data sets were analyzed with T tests/Analysis of Variance (ANOVA) depending on the data sets, utilizing IBM SPSS statistics software (Version 28.0.0.0) [23]. The "alpha level" was set as 0.05 for the analyses ($\alpha = 0.05$).

3. Results

The demographic information of the 12 participants was reviewed and is summarized in **Table 1**.

The majority of the participants were male (83.3%), Hispanic (66.7%), nonsmoker (91.7%), and non-veterans (91.7%) with some college education (66.7%). All of them denied any medication use or current medical issues. The average age of the 12 participants was 32.9 years old with a range of 20 to 57 years old. The average BMI was 29.1 kg/m^2 with a range of 21 to 40.3 kg/m^2.

The "naloxone" and "creatinine" levels were checked, and the average and standard deviation (SD) of the four different specimen aliquots in each sample are listed in **Table 2**. The "naloxone" level with maximum measurable level was 1000 ng/mL, and any values surpassing it were considered as 1000 ng/mL for the purpose of calculations. Similarly, when the "naloxone" level was lower than the minimal measurable or detectable level (<100 ng/mL), 0 ng/mL was used for the purpose of calculations. The reportable range of "creatinine" was 5-2239 mg/dL, while that of "naloxone" was 100-1000 ng/mL. The "naloxone" was reported with the unit of ng/mL while that of "creatinine" with mg/dL.

Table 2 shows that when buprenorphine/naloxone film was dipped directly into these specimens, "naloxone" was detected in the samples. Although "naloxone" was not detected in one of the 1 mm*3 sec specimens, all of the other specimens had "naloxone" detected in the urine specimens. In particular, all of the specimens with full film dipped for 30 seconds showed high levels of "naloxone" detected with >1000 ng/mL. All the creatinine levels were within normal range (20–400 mg/dL in the ARUP laboratory report) with an average of 89.75 mg/dL.

A statistically significant difference is present when we compared with 1 mm dipped for 3 seconds, half film dipped for 3 seconds, and full film dipped for 3 seconds by a one-way ANOVA ($F(2, 33) = [3.401]$, $p = .045$). This indicates that the larger the area of film in contact with the urine specimen, the higher the level of "naloxone" detected in the urine. Also, when we compare the specimens that had a full film dipped for 3 seconds ($M = 765.83$, $SD = 356.91$) versus 30 seconds ($M = 1000$,

Characteristic (N = 12)	Mean ± SD or n (%)	Range
Age (y)	32.9 ± 11.3	20–57
Sex, Male	10 (83.3.%)	
Ethnicity	8 (66.7%)	
Hispanic	3 (25%)	
White Other	1 (8.3%)	
BMI (kg/m^2)	29.1 ± 5.7	21–40.3
Smoking		
Never	11 (91.7%)	
Smoker	1 (8.3%)	
Veterans	1 (8.3%)	
Education		
Some college	8 (66.7%)	
Bachelor's	3 (25%)	
Others	1 (8.3%)	

The information is presented as mean ± standard deviation (SD) or mean with n (number) in %. BMI, body mass index.

Table 1.
Demographic information of 12 participants.

Subjects	Aliquot 1 (1 mm*3 sec)	Aliquot 2 (half*3 sec)	Aliquot 3 (full*3 sec)	Aliquot 4 (full*30 sec)	Creatinine mg/dL
1	<100	337	>1000	>1000	84
2	331	>1000	>1000	>1000	165
3	>1000	110	117	>1000	52
4	407	>1000	>1000	>1000	27
5	933	>1000	>1000	>1000	159
6	226	>1000	>1000	>1000	45
7	809	>1000	>1000	>1000	97
8	233	>1000	>1000	>1000	67
9	524	>1000	>1000	>1000	75
10	187	969	504	>1000	138
11	263	601	354	>1000	73
12	991	>1000	215	>1000	95
Average	492.00	834.75	765.83	1000.00	89.75
SD	351.82	311.03	356.91	0.00	43.98

*Aliquot 1 (1 mm*3 sec) = a buprenorphine/naloxone film was dipped vertically 1 mm for three seconds; Aliquot 2 (half*3 sec) = half film was dipped for three seconds; Aliquot 3 (full*3 sec) = full film was dipped for three seconds; and Aliquot 4 (full*30 sec) = full film was dipped for 30 seconds. SD = Standard Deviation.*

Table 2.
"Naloxone" levels in 12 urine samples.

SD = 0) by an independent sample T test, a statistically significant difference of "naloxone" levels was observed; t(22) = −2.273, p = .033). This indicates the longer the time the film was dipped, the higher the "naloxone" levels were detected. Thus, these results indicate that the volume and duration of dipping can influence "naloxone" levels in urine.

Next, the average of "naloxone" levels in the 12 urine specimens, the diluted 10% urine sample, and purified water sample were compared. The results are summarized in **Table 3**. In the table below, "naloxone", "creatinine" and "naloxone/creatinine" levels are listed with the units and the cut off levels. Because the unit of "naloxone" was recorded with "ng/mL" while that of "creatinine" was (mg/dL), the ratio between "naloxone" and "creatinine" was listed with ($*^{-4}$) for an easier understanding.

Table 3 shows that when the film was dipped into purified water without human urine, "naloxone" was detected. This indicates that "naloxone" detected in urine might be mere dissolvents instead of metabolites. Next, the "naloxone" levels of room

Samples		"Naloxone" ng/mL (100–1000)	"Creatinine" mg/dL (5–2239)	"Naloxone"/"Creatinine" ($*^{-4}$)
Water BT	1 mm*3 sec	637	ND	NA
	Half*3 sec	>1000	ND	NA
	Full*3 sec	>1000	ND	NA
	Full*30 sec	>1000	ND	NA
Water RT	1 mm*3 sec	347	ND	NA
	Half*3 sec	>1000	ND	NA
	Full*3 sec	>1000	ND	NA
	Full*30 sec	>1000	ND	NA
10% BT	1 mm*3 sec	304	7	43.43
	Half*3 sec	>1000	7	142.86
	Full*3 sec	468	7	66.86
	Full*30 sec	>1000	7	142.86
10% RT	1 mm*3 sec	ND	6	NA
	Half*3 sec	761	6	126.83
	Full*3 sec	436	6	72.67
	Full*30 sec	>1000	6	166.67
Urine BT	1 mm*3 sec	492	89.75	6.78
(12 urine	Half*3 sec	834.75	89.75	11.84
average)	Full*3 sec	765.83	89.75	11.26
	Full*30 sec	>1000	89.75	14.4

ND (not detected) indicates that the "naloxone" or "creatinine" was under the detectable level. NA (not applicable) indicates that "naloxone" or "creatinine" was undetected, and thus we were not able to calculate "naloxone"/"creatinine" ratio. BT (body temperature) means that the sample temperature was ~97° F. RT (room temperature) in 10% RT means that the samples were diluted by room temperature purified water. The unit as well as the minimal and maximal measurable levels are listed in the table. "Creatinine" levels of four specimens in one sample are the same because only one urine "creatinine" level in each sample was tested.

Table 3.
"Naloxone" levels in urine specimens, 10% diluted urine, and purified water.

temperature water were compared with those of body temperature with one-sample T-test. We found that the "naloxone" levels of room temperature water ($M = 836.75$, $SD = 326.50$) were not significantly different from those with body temperature water ($M = 909.25$, $SD = 181.50$); $t(6) = .388$, $p = .711$). Thus, the temperature difference did not affect "naloxone" levels. Finally, when the "naloxone" levels of body temperature purified water, body temperature 10% urine and body temperature pure urine were compared by a one-way ANOVA, there was no statistical difference ($F(2, 9) = [.690]$, $p = .526$). Thus, the urine concentration difference did not affect "naloxone" levels. These results indicate that temperature and concentration of urine samples did not affects "naloxone" levels.

4. Discussion

4.1 Clinical effects of sublingual naloxone

This study demonstrated that high levels of "naloxone" were found in adulterated urine samples from individuals who were not taking any medications. High levels of "naloxone" were also detected in the purified water samples when buprenorphine/naloxone film was dipped into the samples. Thus, these results and those in the previous studies on urine "naloxone" levels suggest that "naloxone" can be detected in adulterated urine samples both from those who are not on buprenorphine/naloxone and those who are on buprenorphine/naloxone [15, 20]. This information can lead to the speculation that "naloxone" detected in urine samples can be mere dissolvents of some fraction of naloxone instead of metabolites, and consequently imply a possibility that "naloxone" in urine samples from the patients taking buprenorphine/naloxone films were the mere dissolvents of some naloxone in the urinary system, considering naloxone's low bioavailability and extensive first-pass metabolism. Unfortunately, we were unable to distinguish between "naloxone" in urine that has been excreted by nephrons after it was absorbed and metabolized versus some fractions of "naloxone" that have been only dissolved in the system.

The clinical effects of sublingual naloxone on healthy patients have been controversial. For example, Nasser, et al. conducted a research study, in which 43 participants received one single sublingual tablet of brand name Suboxone (buprenorphine/naloxone 2 mg/0.5 mg) and their plasma "naloxone" levels in their blood samples were monitored for up to 168 hours. They found that the participants with severe hepatic impairment had higher and longer "naloxone" levels detected compared with the healthy participants; however, the inactive metabolite, "naloxone 3-β-D-glucuronide" levels were similar between the two groups. They concluded that sublingual buprenorphine/naloxone combined product should be avoided for those who have severe hepatic impairment [4]. This study also suggested that naloxone is metabolized in the liver and may provide clinical effectiveness only for those who have hepatic impairment. The clinical effects of sublingual naloxone on healthy patients remain controversial.

Strickland and Burson reviewed the charts of 561 patients, 11.1% of whom were on buprenorphine/naloxone combination products while the others received mono products. The authors reported that urine "naloxone" was detected in the majority of samples; 97.8% from the 63 patients who were on the dual medication had >1 ng/mL naloxone, and 92.7% of them had 30 ng/mL of naloxone. The authors argued that sublingual naloxone may be absorbed and thus cause unpleasant adverse effects [13].

By contrast, the pharmacological effects of sublingual naloxone have a 10-times lower binding affinity to μ opioid receptors, compared to buprenorphine, namely, rapid opioid receptor dissociation (approximately 6.5 minutes); short half-life of naloxone (60–90 minutes compared to 24–60 hours of buprenorphine); low bioavailability (estimated 3% sublingually); and first-pass bioavailablility, led to the postulation of insignificant clinical effects in sublingual naloxone. After the Food and Drug Administration (FDA) approved buprenorphine/naloxone combination medication in 2002 [24], this combined medication became the standard of care, especially after the Substance Abuse and Mental Health Services Administration (SAMHSA) warned about the misuse potentials of monotherapy [25]. However, the controversy of combined naloxone/buprenorphine versus monotherapy of buprenorphine has yet to be resolved, and further research and discussion on this topic await.

4.2 Adulteration

This study found that the amount of the film that was used to adulterated urine specimen did affect the concentration of "naloxone" detected in the urine. Submerging a small portion of the film for a short period of time (1 mm*3 sec) in this study resulted in an average of 492 ng/mL of "naloxone" levels in the urine samples among the 12 participants. By contrast, the urine samples with full film dipped into the aliquot for 3 seconds (Full*3 sec) yielded an average of 765.83 ng/mL of "naloxone". These numbers are very similar with those found in the study done by Warrington, et al. on the "naloxone" levels in suspected adulterated urine. They retrospectively reviewed "naloxone" levels of 1223 urine samples from two practice sites and reported that the average "naloxone" level was "633.65ng/mL (range 1-12,161 ng/mL) with 54% of samples <300 ng/mL and 8.0% having >2000ng/mL. One of the sites had increased evidence of urine adulteration and 9.3% of the samples from this site contained > 2000 ng/ml of "naloxone" with an average of 686.8 ng/mL. The other site had no report of urine adulteration and demonstrated an average "naloxone" level of 570.9 ng/mL with 6.4% of samples containing > 2000 ng/mL. This study concluded that extremely high levels of "naloxone" can suggest urine adulteration [20]. Furo also reviewed 97 patient charts with urine drug screening results in an outpatient telemedicine OUD clinic and found that average "naloxone" level was 687.2 ng/mL that ranged from 5 ng/mL to>2000 ng/mL with 15.30% >2000 ng/mL [26].

Heikman, et al. collected 40 urine samples from 32 patients and found much lower average of "naloxone" levels in their study. In their study design, the first group (Group 0: pre-treatment) received parental buprenorphine before buprenorphine/naloxone treatment; the second group (Group 1: stable patients) consisted of stable patients who were on prescribed sublingual buprenorphine/naloxone treatment without any illicit substances in their urine; and the third group (Group 2: unstable patients) had prescribed sublingual buprenorphine/naloxone with unexpected urine test results. The urine samples were collected about 24 hours after the last buprenorphine/naloxone medication dispensation. The study found that the median naloxone level in the stable phase was 60 μg/L (=ng/mL, henceforth ng/mL), ranged from 5 ng/mL to 200 ng/mL while that in the unstable phase was 70 ng/mL, ranged from 70 ng/mL to 1700 ng/mL. They concluded that high "naloxone" level can indicate non-compliance of buprenorphine/naloxone treatment [15].

The average "naloxone" levels in the study by Heikman, et al., [15] was much lower compared with those in the studies mentioned above. This may be because naloxone has a short half-life of 60–90 minutes [22] and because their urine collection was done approximately 24 hours after the last dose of buprenorphine/naloxone medication. The average "naloxone" levels of this current study (e.g. 492 ng/mL of 1 mm*3 sec specimen group and 765.83 ng/mL of full*3 sec group) of the adulterated urine samples from those who were not on buprenorphine/naloxone were similar to those of these previous studies (e.g. 687.2 ng/mL in Furo [26] and 570.9 ng/mL in Warrington, et al. [20]) with the unadulterated urine samples from those were on buprenorphine/naloxone. This similarity should be explored further in relation to the implication of pharmacokinetics and pharmacodynamics of naloxone in the system.

4.3 Clinical applications

The results of this study can be used to help clinicians interpret urine toxicology test results more accurately. In this section, seven simulated cases based on previously encountered results are discussed to present how to apply the findings of this study to the daily practice of OUD treatment. The cases and their associated laboratory values as well as the buprenorphine prescription dosage are summarized in **Table 4**.

4.3.1 Case 1

[Bup 278 ng/mL, Norbup 635 ng/mL, Bup/Norbup 0.44, Nal 687 ng/mL, Cre 133.9 mg/dL, Bup/Nal 16 mg/4 mg per day, appropriate case].

This is a typical pattern of urine toxicology results. If patients are taking "buprenorphine" daily, "norbuprenorphine" is usually higher than "buprenorphine", [16] and creatinine is within normal range (20-400 mg/dL) (The ARUP laboratory criteria). Therefore, this is an appropriate urine toxicology case for those who are compliant with buprenorphine/naloxone treatment.

4.3.2 Case 2

[Bup >2000 ng/mL, Norbup 17 ng/mL, Bup/Norbup 117.65, Nal >2000 ng/mL, Cre 97.2 mg/dL, Bup/Nal 16 mg/4 mg per day, inappropriate case].

Cases	Bup (ng/mL)	Norbup (ng/mL)	Bup/ Norbup	Nal (ng/mL)	Cre (mg/dL)	Bup /nal prescription (dose per day)
Case 1	278	635	0.44	687	133.9	Bup/Nal 16 mg/4 mg
Case 2	>2000	17	117.65	>2000	97.2	Bup/Nal 16 mg/4 mg
Case 3	>2000	>2000	1.00	>2000	306.7	Bup/Nal 16 mg/4 mg
Case 4	>2000	10	200.00	<2 (undetectable)	82.6	Bup 16 mg
Case 5	>2000	17	117.65	5	179.2	Bup/Nal 16 mg/4 mg
Case 6	>2000	>2000	1.00	>2000	82.5	Bup/Nal 16 mg/4 mg
Case 7	286	569	0.50	71	67.5	Bup 16 mg

Bup = Buprenorphine, Norbup = Norbuprenorphine, Nal = Naloxone, Cre = Creatinine. The units are listed in the top column. The level > 2000 ng/mL was considered 2000 ng/mL for the calculations.

Table 4.
7 simulated cases in clinical practice and their associated laboratory values.

This is a typical pattern of urine adulteration of having dipped buprenorphine/naloxone film directly into the urine sample. The ratio between buprenorphine/norbuprenorphine is >50 [17]. The very high naloxone level (>2000 ng/mL) confirms this suspicion of adulteration, consistent with the results of this study.

4.3.3 Case 3

[Bup >2000 ng/mL, Norbup >2000 ng/mL, Bup/Norbup 1.0, Nal >2000 ng/mL, Cre 306.7 mg, Bup/Nal 16 mg/4 mg per day, appropriate case].

This case has a high level of naloxone >2000 ng/mL, so there is suspicion of urine adulteration; however, this is an example, in which a high naloxone level does not mean urine adulteration. As Furo's study found that 15% of urine samples had "naloxone" levels >2000 ng/mL [26], a high level of naloxone can also be due to other reasons. This case illustrates that we can use a high "naloxone" level to confirm urine adulteration only if the buprenorphine/naloxone ratio is >50:1; "naloxone" level itself cannot be the main determining factor of urine adulteration. In other words, the judgment of urine adulteration should be based on high buprenorphine/norbuprenorphine ratio. Therefore, this is an appropriate case of buprenorphine/naloxone treatment. One might wonder why is this patient's "naloxone" level so high? The answer is that this patient might be dehydrated at the time of this urine collection, indicated by the high creatinine level, so the buprenorphine, norbuprenorphine, naloxone and creatinine are all consequently very high. If this patient were well hydrated, the results should have been similar to Case 1 with a much lower creatinine level. Thus, this example should be appropriate for the buprenorphine/norbuprenorphine treatment.

4.3.4 Case 4

[Bup >2000 ng/mL, Norbup 10 ng/mL, Bup/Norbup 200, Nal <2 ng/mL, Cre 82.6 mg/dL, Bup 16 mg per day, inappropriate case].

This case is an adulteration case in which the patient is prescribed buprenorphine only medication. This patient has not taken this medication for a while, indicated by the low norbuprenorphine level. This case has a high ratio of buprenorphine/norbuprenorphine, but naloxone is undetectable, which means that prior to the urine collection, buprenorphine medication has been crushed into powder and dissolved into the sample. As a result, the ratio between buprenorphine/norbuprenorphine is high (>50), but there is undetectable naloxone level (<2 ng/mL). Undetectable naloxone level should be always suspected with buprenorphine monotherapy.

4.3.5 Case 5

[Bup >2000 ng/mL, Norbup 17 ng/mL, Bup/Norbup 117.65, Nal 5 ng/mL, Cre 179.2 mg/dL, Bup/Nal 16 mg/4 mg per day, inappropriate case].

This is another case of urine adulteration as indicated with a high buprenorphine/norbuprenorphine ratio (>50:1). However, "naloxone" is detected at a very small amount. Because of the high buprenorphine/norbuprenorphine ratio, we expect a high level of "naloxone" if buprenorphine/naloxone was dipped in this urine sample. Otherwise, we expect undetectable level of "naloxone" if buprenorphine only medication was dissolved into the urine sample. The small amount of "naloxone's being detected means that this patient probably has taken buprenorphine/naloxone at least 24 hours before this urine collection [15], and thus there was a small amount of "naloxone" residue detected. Compared with buprenorphine, the naloxone's half-life is much shorter, and thus, a low level of naloxone can be detected while relatively higher level of buprenorphine and norbuprenorphine still remained in the system after an intermittent use of buprenorphine/naloxone. In addition, this patient tampered the urine sample with buprenorphine only medication, which is indicated by the high buprenorphine/norbuprenorphine ratio. If buprenorphine/naloxone combined medication was dipped into this urine sample, the naloxone level would have been much higher as indicated by the results of this study, unless the patient has some issues of naloxone metabolism such as the enzyme to metabolize naloxone is inhibited by certain medication(s) or genetically. This patient is prescribed with buprenorphine/naloxone combined medication, so it is uncertain as to why this patient added additional buprenorphine to the urine.

4.3.6 Case 6

[Bup >2000 ng/mL, Norbup 2000 ng/mL, Bup/Norbup 1.0, Nal 2000 ng/mL, Cre 82.5 mg/dL, Bup/Nal 16 mg/4 mg per day, appropriate case].

This case has high "buprenorphine", "norbuprenorphine" and "naloxone" levels, so we can speculate dehydration; however, "creatinine" level is not as high as Case 3, and therefore, we can rule out dehydration. The ratio between buprenorphine to norbuprenorphine is <50:1, so it is unlikely that this sample is adulterated. This might be a case with high metabolism patient, which causes high levels of all components. This is rare but can happen. Thus, this is another example of a high naloxone level, but it does not mean urine adulteration.

4.3.7 Case 7

[Bup 286 ng/mL, Norbup 569 ng/mL, Bup/Norbup 0.5, Nal 71 ng/mL, Cre 67.5 mg/dL, Bup 16 mg per day due to naloxone allergies, inappropriate case].

This patient has an appropriate "buprenorphine" to "norbuprenorphine" ratio (<50:1) with low level of "naloxone"; however, this result is not appropriate because this patient was on buprenorphine monotherapy due to naloxone allergies. The detected "naloxone" suggests that she has been taking buprenorphine/naloxone despite her being prescribed buprenorphine monotherapy. Buprenorphine only product has a higher street value than buprenorphine/norbuprenorphine combined medication by approximately 20% [27]. Therefore, some patients might trade their buprenorphine with buprenorphine/naloxone combination medication for the marginal profit.

In summary, as this study found, a high concentration of "naloxone" can confirm suspected urine adulteration if buprenorphine/norbuprenorphine ratio is >50:1. However, a high level of "naloxone" alone does not necessarily involve urine adulteration, especially without a high ratio of buprenorphine/norbuprenorphine. The patient might have dehydrated at the time of urine collection, or the patient might be a fast metabolizer of buprenorphine/naloxone. Therefore, we should monitor creatinine level because it can indicate the hydration status of the patient [28], as dehydration can cause high levels of "naloxone" in addition to high "buprenorphine" and "norbuprenorphine" levels. Furthermore, a patient with high metabolism can cause high levels of "buprenorphine", "norbuprenorphine" and "naloxone" without a corresponding high "creatinine" level. Finally, if "naloxone" is observed in urine sample, we can suspect that the patient is taking or had taken buprenorphine/naloxone combined medication, while if no naloxone is identified, the patient is on buprenorphine monotherapy.

4.4 Clinical implications

The results of this study have implications on clinical practice in the care of OUD patients. With the increased use of unobserved urine toxicology collection in practice [29], the appropriate interpretation of urine drug tests remains a challenging but vital component of comprehensive patient care. Results from this study may suggest that the "naloxone" detected in adulterated urine samples may be dissolved "naloxone" instead of metabolized naloxone, or a fraction of naloxone at least. There are also healthcare policy implications with the controversy of mono-product formulation use in the United States as a harm reduction approach in the treatment of OUD [9]. Buprenorphine mono-product is used widely in other areas of the world [30] and has been suggested as a medication treatment option for patients struggling with adverse effects, thought to be potentially from naloxone absorption from sublingual buprenorphine/naloxone combined medication [9]. With increasing research findings that raise the concern of using "naloxone" levels in urine as an indicator of absorption of naloxone and potentially the cause of patient-reported adverse effects, these findings reinforce the recommendation for clinicians to also consider possible urine adulteration, resulting in elevated "naloxone" levels.

A high level of "naloxone" itself should trigger further assessment of the patient buprenorphine/naloxone regimen; however, by itself there is insufficient evidence to guide care. This information should be synthesized with other available urine toxicology screen parameters (buprenorphine, norbuprenorphine, creatinine and buprenorphine/norbuprenorphine ratio) to better inform the clinical picture. Moreover, the continuation of buprenorphine as a medication for OUD yields more benefits than risks in the public health approach of addressing opioid overdose mortality. Urine toxicology is only one piece of information to be used in a clinical evaluation. The overall goal of improvement of multiple biopsychosocial domains and patient-centered outcomes remains the driving force in clinical decision-making.

Finally, the results of this study might support the stipulation that sublingual naloxone can be minimally absorbed and metabolized in the system and thus exerts insignificant effects clinically when taken sublingually, which might consequently contribute to the controversy on buprenorphine/naloxone combined product versus buprenorphine monotherapy in the buprenorphine induction process [31, 32]. The results of this study would give us an insight on these controversial issues.

4.5 Limitations

The limitations of this study include the small sample size and reliance on subjects' report of substance and medication use. Findings from this study may be used to apply for funding to support a larger sample size study and additional substance testing of all samples. While the potential effects of unreported substance use are unknown, the overall trend in this study's results is unlikely to be impacted. An additional limitation is that this study evaluated the addition of varying buprenorphine/naloxone levels via film into water and urine samples as a proxy for adulteration. The actual adulteration techniques used by individuals may vary widely. A clinical trial evaluating "naloxone" levels in adulterated and non-adulterated urine samples of patients prescribed buprenorphine/naloxone would be difficult in nature. To address the range in adulteration techniques, we used multiple categories of surface areas, dipping duration, temperatures, and concentrations of both urine and water samples to assimilate a variety of methods and observe the resulting "naloxone" levels. Finally, we also acknowledge that some clinicians use urine toxicology that do not report "naloxone" levels in certain clinic practices, and therefore these findings may not be clinically useful to all providers.

5. Conclusions

The urine "naloxone" level by dissolving buprenorphine/naloxone film is very sensitive to the area and the time that the film come into contact with the urine samples. Attempted adulteration of the urine sample is likely yield supratherapeutic levels of "naloxone". At this time, there is no consensus as to what level to set the "naloxone" concentration as a parameter to determine the legitimacy of patient urine samples except some research reports. While "naloxone" level is a simple component to test for in resource-challenged practices, other metabolites such as "buprenorphine" and its metabolite levels should be examined to guide clinical decisions. In summary, the results of this study have provided a further insight into interpreting urine drug screening test results for OUD patients with buprenorphine treatment. Strict monitoring of urine toxicology is by no means a punitive process but to improve the outcome of OUD treatment. Future study can focus on differentiating naloxone molecules that were dissolved "naloxone" versus those that were renally excreted, which can enhance our understanding on the pharmacokinetics and pharmacodynamics of naloxone.

Acknowledgements

We would like to express our sincere and deep appreciation for the editors and reviewers who provided us with valuable feedback. We would also thank Editage for editing the final version of this manuscript.

Authors' contributions

H.F. carried out the research experiment and wrote the first draft of the paper excerpt discussion and conclusion sections. T.H. wrote the discussion and conclusion sections and completed the manuscript with support with S.A. who edited the draft form of this manuscript. Y.Z. completed the manuscript by editing the final version.

Funding

Not applicable.

Competing interests

There is no conflict of interests among the authors.

Consent for publication

All authors agree with publishing this manuscript.

Note

Correspondence concerning this article should be addressed to Hiroko Furo (furo@uthscsa.edu), Department of Psychiatry and Behavioral Sciences, the University of Texas Health at San Antonio, San Antonio, TX, USA.

Ethics approval and consent to participate

The Institutional Review Board (IRB) application to the University of Texas Health at San Antonio was approved (IRB Protocol ID: 20220593HU), and the written consents were obtained by all participants.

Availability of data and materials

The datasets produced for the data analysis for this study are not publicly available due to the confidentiality of participants but are available in a de-identified form from the corresponding author on request.

Abbreviations

"Naloxone" levels in 12 urine samples—1 mm*3 sec	buprenorphine/naloxone film was dipped vertically 1 mm for three seconds
Half*3 sec	half film was dipped for three seconds
Full*3 sec	full film was dipped for three seconds
Full*30 sec	full film was dipped for 30 seconds
RT	room temperature
BT	body temperature ~ 97°F
ND	not detected
SD	standard deviation
N	number
BMI	body mass index
M	mean

Author details

Hiroko Furo[1,2,3,4*], Tony Lin[4], Yi Yuan Zhou[2] and Sarah Abdelsayed[4]

1 Department of Psychiatry and Behavioral Sciences, The University of Texas Health at San Antonio, San Antonio, TX, USA

2 Department of Pathology, The University of Texas Health at San Antonio, San Antonio, TX, USA

3 Department of Biomedical Informatics, State University of New York (SUNY) at Buffalo, Buffalo, NY, USA

4 Department of Family Medicine, State University of New York (SUNY) at Buffalo, Buffalo, NY, USA

*Address all correspondence to: hfuro1@gmail.com

References

[1] "Naloxone". Drugbank Online. 11/28/22. https://go.drugbank.com/drugs/DB01183

[2] Koyyalagunta D. Opioid analgesics. In: Pain Management. Netherlands: Elsevier; 2007. pp. 939-964

[3] Jordan MR, Morrisonponce D. Naloxone. In: StatPearls [Internet]. Treasure Island (FL): StatPearls Publishing; 2022. Available from: https://www.ncbi.nlm.nih.gov/books/NBK441910/ . [Accessed: Jul 11, 2022]

[4] Nasser AF, Heidbreder C, Liu Y, et al. Pharmacokinetics of sublingual buprenorphine and naloxone in subjects with mild to severe hepatic impairment (child-pugh classes A, B, and C), in hepatitis C virus-seropositive subjects, and in healthy volunteers. Clinical Pharmacokinetics. 2015;**54**:837-849. DOI: 10.1007/s40262-015-0238-6

[5] Coe MA, Lofwall MR, Walsh SL. Buprenorphine pharmacology review: Update on transmucosal and long-acting formulations. Journal of Addiction Medicine. 2019;**13**(2):93-103. DOI: 10.1097/ADM.0000000000000457

[6] Available from: https://www.fda.gov/media/100429/download#:~:text=Naloxone%20is%20absorbed%20not%20only,is%20within%201%2D2%20minutes

[7] Preston KL, Bigelow GE, Liebson IA. Effects of sublingually given naloxone in opioid-dependent human volunteers. Drug and Alcohol Dependence. 1990;*25*(1):27-34. DOI: 10.1016/0376-8716(90)90136-3

[8] NIDA. Naloxone DrugFacts. National Institute on Drug Abuse website. 2022 Available from: https://nida.nih.gov/publications/drugfacts/naloxone [Accessed: November 26, 2022]

[9] Blazes CK, Morrow JD. Reconsidering the usefulness of adding naloxone to buprenorphine. Frontiers in Psychiatry. 2020;**11**:549272. DOI: 10.3389/fpsyt.2020.549272

[10] Mendelson J, Jones RT, Welm S, et al. Buprenorphine and naloxone combinations: the effects of three dose ratios in morphine-stabilized, opiate-dependent volunteers. Psychopharmacology. 1999;**141**(1):37-46. DOI: 10.1007/s002130050804

[11] Tzatzarakis MN, Vakonaki E, Kovatsi L, et al. Determination of buprenorphine, norbuprenorphine and naloxone in fingernail clippings and urine of patients under opioid substitution therapy. Journal of Analytical Toxicology. 2015;**39**(4):313-320

[12] Stone, JA Pesce AJ, Fitzgerald RL. 2017 Fake news, alternative facts or just normal pharmacokinetics? High urine naloxone concentrations in patients prescribed sublingual buprenorphine–naloxone (BNX). MSACL EU Abstract

[13] Strickland DM, Burson JK. Sublingual absorption of naloxone in a large clinical population. Journal of Drug Metabolic Toxicology. 2018;**09**(02):1-4

[14] Rosado J, Walsh SL, Bigelow GE, Strain EC. Sublingual buprenorphine/naloxone precipitated withdrawal in subjects maintained on 100mg of daily methadone. Drug and Alcohol Dependence. 2007;**90**(2-3):261-269. DOI: 10.1016/j.drugalcdep.2007.04.006

[15] Heikman P, Häkkinen M, Gergov M, Ojanperä I. Urine naloxone concentration

at different phases of buprenorphine maintenance treatment: Urine naloxone concentration at buprenorphine maintenance treatment. Drug Test Analysis. 2014;**6**(3):220-225

[16] Furo H, Schwartz DG, Sullivan RW, Elkin PL. Buprenorphine dosage and urine quantitative buprenorphine, norbuprenorphine, and creatinine levels in an office-based opioid treatment program. Substance Abuse. 2021;**15**:1-9 11782218211061749. DOI: 10.1177/11782218211061749

[17] Accurso AJ, Lee JD, McNeely J. High prevalence of urine tampering in an office-based opioid treatment practice detected by evaluating the norbuprenorphine to buprenorphine ratio. Journal of Substance Abuse Treatment. 2017;**83**:62-67. DOI: 10.1016/j.jsat.2017.10.002

[18] Donroe JH, Holt SR, O'Connor PG, Sukumar N, Tetrault JM. Interpreting quantitative urine buprenorphine and norbuprenorphine levels in office-based clinical practice. Drug and Alcohol Dependence. 2017;**180**:46-51. DOI: 10.1016/j.drugalcdep.2017.07.040

[19] Suzuki J, Zinser J, Issa M, Rodriguez C. Quantitative testing of buprenorphine and norbuprenorphine to identify urine sample spiking during office-based opioid treatment. Substance Abuse. 2017;**38**(4):504-507. DOI: 10.1080/08897077.2017.1356796

[20] Warrington JS, Booth K, Warrington GS, et al. Use of urinary naloxone levels in a single provider practice: a case study. Addiction Science & Clinical Practice. 2020;**15**:3. DOI: 10.1186/s13722-020-0178-9

[21] Burns MM, Law TC, Rifai N, Shannon MW. Naloxone produces a positive urine opiate screen. Pediatric Research. 1999;**45**(7):80-80

[22] Clarke SFJ, Dargan PI, Jones AL. Naloxone in opioid poisoning: Walking the tightrope. Emergency Medicine Journal. 2005;**22**:612-616

[23] Available from: https://www.ibm.com/spss

[24] "Buprenorphine". Drug enforcement administration—diversion control division: Drug and chemical evaluation section. 11/28/22. Available from: https://www.deadiversion.usdoj.gov/drug_chem_info/buprenorphine.pdf

[25] Walsh L. Buprenorphine. Available from: https://www.samhsa.gov/medication-assisted-treatment/treatment/buprenorphine,

[26] "Interpretation of urine drug test results of buprenorphine, norbuprenorphine, naloxone, creatinine levels in buprenorphine treatment program. Work-in-Progress. Furo H.

[27] Hswen Y, Zhang A, Brownstein JS. Leveraging black-market street buprenorphine pricing to increase capacity to treat opioid addiction, 2010-2018. Preventive Medicine. 2020;**137**:106105. DOI: 10.1016/j.ypmed.2020.106105

[28] Weigand TJ, editor. Use and interpretation of buprenorphine metabolite profiles during maintenance treatment. In: Poster Presented at: 47th American Society of Addiction Medicine (ASAM) Annual Conference, April 14-17. MD: Baltimore; 2016

[29] Rao PN, Jotwani R, Joshi J, Gulati A, Mehta N. Reevaluating chronic opioid monitoring during and after the COVID-19 pandemic. Pain Management. 2020;**10**(6):353-358. DOI: 10.2217/pmt-2020-0063

[30] Yokell MA, Zaller ND, Green TC, Rich JD. Buprenorphine and

buprenorphine/naloxone diversion, misuse, and illicit use: an international review. Current Drug Abuse Reviews. 2011;**4**(1):28-41. DOI: 10.2174/1874473711104010028

[31] Rzasa Lynn R, Galinkin JL. Naloxone dosage for opioid reversal: current evidence and clinical implications. Therory of Advanced Drug Safety. 2018;**9**(1):63-88. DOI: 10.1177/2042098617744161

[32] Dooley J, Gerber-Finn L, Antone I, Guilfoyle J, Blakelock B, Balfour-Boehm J, et al. Buprenorphine-naloxone use in pregnancy for treatment of opioid dependence: Retrospective cohort study of 30 patients. Canadian Family Physician. 2016;**62**(4):e194-e200

Chapter 7

Usefulness of Urine Tests in the Prevention, Diagnosis, Treatment and Prognosis of Pathologies Present during Pregnancy

Noren Villalobos

Abstract

Pregnancy produces physiological changes in the woman necessary to be able to bring it to a happy term. However, they can favor the development of pathologies in various organs and systems, ranging from urinary infections, diabetes mellitus or gestational to hypertensive disorders of pregnancy. Which produce substances that are excreted through the urine. There is also excretion of metabolites which can be evaluated for the diagnosis and prognosis of certain chromosomopathies. These substances, when measured or quantified, provide bases for diagnosis, prevention, and allow decisions to be made regarding timely treatment in many of them.

Keywords: urinalysis, pregnancy, pathologies of pregnancy, diagnosis, urinary tract infections

1. Introduction

Pregnancy (EMB) is considered a physiological state where the maternal organism must adapt to the allograft it carries in its body [1]. To do this, it undergoes a series of modifications or physiological changes that allow it to adapt to the EMB in a continuous and dynamic way, which occur at the level of all organs and systems, and in turn are influenced by multiple factors that include the age of the woman, previous pregnancies, physical and nutritional status, presence of previous diseases or pathologies, among others [2]. These changes regress after the birth of the fetus in a period of approximately 40 days or until the moment the menstrual cycle resumes, returning the mother to the state prior to pregnancy and preparing her body for a new pregnancy [1, 2].

These changes known as gravid or physiological modifications of pregnancy (MFE) can be monitored through laboratory tests and diagnostic aid images (such as ultrasound) which can be routinely performed quarterly in normal EMB or vary their frequency in those cases in which complications or pathologies associated with it appear, which are capable of modifying its course or aggravating or unmasking a pre-existing problem [3].

1.1 MFEs comprise

a. Changes observable by the mother that are capable of producing specific symptoms such as weight gain, abdominal volume increase, breast growth, frequency, constipation, vaginal discharge, heartburn, skin hyperpigmentation [2].

b. Changes that can be assessed through physical examination by health personnel, such as blood pressure, changes in heart rate, changes in respiratory rate, and the presence of a noise in S3 on auscultation [2].

c. Changes detected through diagnostic aid studies in images such as basic ultrasound or the use of Doppler and through laboratory tests that include hematology, blood chemistry, serology and urinalysis or urine test [2].

The kidney is one of the organs that undergo important changes with the EMB which begin from the 6th week beginning with anatomical changes that include dilation of the pelvis and renal calyces and ureters, all this under the action of pregnancy hormones. Progesterone and estrogens [1, 2]. This causes an increase in urinary dead space, at the same time that renal vascularization increases with an increase in interstitial volume, which in turn causes an increase in kidney length of approximately 1 to 1.5 cm. compared to a normal adult (4.5). The kidney recovers its normal size approximately 6 months postpartum, even when the puerperium has already ended.

All of this leads to changes in renal physiology from the hemodynamic point of view, glomerular filtration, water and electrolyte management, and changes in the renin-angiotensin-aldosterone system [4].

A predisposition to the appearance of urinary tract infections (UI) occurs due to compression of the right ureter by dextrorotation of the uterus, to which the sigmoid colon contributes, which compresses the right ureter, and to the decrease in its peristalsis due to the action of progesterone, which favors the appearance of hydronephrosis. in the right kidney, slowing of urine transit through the ureter causing retrograde stasis. Contributing to this is the fact of the residual presence of urine in the urinary bladder, with a decrease in its tone, and a relative increase in its capacity as the EMB progresses due to uterine compression, which even produces reflux into the ureter, and may be up to be for 24 hours or more without being eliminated properly. Its mucosa becomes hyperemic and edematous, making it susceptible to infections and trauma [4].

Renal blood flow increases between 35 and 60%, therefore glomerular filtration increases between 50 and 60% together with the reabsorption of water and electrolytes to maintain the hydroelectrolytic balance [4–6].

During EMB, amino acids and water-soluble vitamins are lost in greater amounts than in non-EMB. Creatinine and uric acid decrease so that normal values for pregnant women are considered normal at 0.8 mgrs.%, and a greater increase is considered suspicious of kidney disease. Creatinine clearance increases by 30%. therefore, values less than 1 37 ml must be evaluated. Glycosuria is not necessarily abnormal and there may be non-significant proteinuria of 115 to 260 mg/day [1].

2. Utilization of urinalysis during pregnancy

2.1 Urinary tract infections

The appearance of urinary tract infections (UTI) is possibly the most frequent pathology during EMB, with a prevalence ranging between 14 and 48% [7], favored by the MFE that occur in the urinary tract and the alkalinization of the urinary tract. Urine [8, 9]. It is associated with other complications of EMB including pyelonephritis, preterm delivery, low birth weight newborns, and increased perinatal mortality [10, 11].

Preterm delivery (PP) is the main complication associated with UTIs, since bacterial infection in maternal and fetal tissues causes the release of endotoxins and exotoxins, cytokines, tumor necrosis factor, interleukin-1 beta, interleukins 6 and 8, granulocyte colony-stimulating factor and other factors, which stimulate the production and release of prostaglandins, leading to uterine contractions and neutrophil activity, which in turn stimulate the synthesis and production of metalloproteinases, causing membrane rupture and collagen remodeling of the cervix [12].

UTI is defined as the presence of 100,000 germs per cubic centimeter (cc) of urine in asymptomatic patients, or greater than 100,000 germs per cc of urine and leukocytes greater than 7 leukocytes per cc of urine in a symptomatic patient [10]. In most cases, it begins in the urinary bladder, favored by MGE, which in turn will allow it to ascend to the kidney [7].

2.1.1 Types of urinary tract infection

Asymptomatic bacteriuria: It is the presence of 100,000 organisms per milliliter (ml) in 2 consecutive cultures with the absence of symptoms, constituting a 40% risk factor for acute cystitis and 25 to 30% for pyelonephritis in pregnancy [9].

UTI: Presence of 100,000 organisms per ml of urine in asymptomatic patients or more than 100,000 accompanied by more than 7 cells in a symptomatic patient [9].

Cystitis: It constitutes the lower UTI characterized by inflammation of the urinary bladder due to bacterial causes or not (radiation) or viral. It occurs in 1 to 2% of pregnant women, being negative in 60% in the first screenings. It is complicated between 15 to 50% with pyelonephritis [9].

Pyelonephritis: upper UTI occurs in approximately 0.5 to 2% of all pregnancies [7, 9].

Now, what should we study in the urine test to help us diagnose UTIs or other pathologies.

2.2 Urinary sediment

The urinary sediment is obtained from a urine sample centrifuged at 2000 revolutions per minute, from which different types of cells originating from the urinary tract epithelium, or other cells such as leukocytes, red blood cells, platelets, renal cells, hyaline casts, are obtained. Leukocyte casts, amorphous phosphates, calcium crystals, uric acid, urates, lipid droplets, cholesterol crystals, proteins [13].

The presence of organisms such as bacteria, which can be typical of the urinary tract or contamination of the vagina, is frequent, as well as protozoa (vaginal trichomonas) and fungi such as candida vaginalis, as well as menstrual products and even spermatozoa [13]. Always contamination vaginal is accompanied by leukocytes and vaginal epithelial cells, so it is necessary to examine the patient's vagina with a speculum when we have these results. Gardnerella vaginalis is another germ that causes infections and vaginal discharges that easily contaminate the urine test.

In the urine analysis, the presence of leucocyte esterase can be evaluated, which is an enzyme secreted by neutrophils, constituting a marker of infection [14, 15]. It has a sensitivity of 83% and a specificity of 78% [16].

Another test used is the nitrite test. It is based on the reduction of nitrates to nitrites carried out by enterobacteria by action of the enzyme nitrite reductase, for which it is necessary that the urine be found without mobilizing for 4 hours, its specificity being that it does not react with other substances [17]. Its sensitivity is 53% and a specificity of 78% [16, 18].

When both studies are combined, they reach a sensitivity of 98% and a specificity of 95%, which makes them very useful in the diagnosis of urinary tract infections [17].

2.3 Ph in urine

The pH of the urine covers the limits of acidity and alkalinity from 5.0 to 8.8. Ph greater than or equal to 6.0 is considered altered [17]. Its determination is a reflection of the buffered ion concentration and not a net measure of acids [18].

Acidic urine, with a pH less than 4.5, may be a reflection of metabolic acidosis, such as diabetic ketoacidosis, which can affect a patient with poorly controlled gestational diabetes or type I or II diabetes during pregnancy. Cases of patients with chronic diarrhea, a diet rich in meat, or in cases of chronic respiratory failure [18].

In contrast, alkaline urine presents with a pH greater than 8.0 and may be due to renal tubular acidosis, metabolic alkalosis which may be caused by pregnancy vomiting in the first trimester or in the case of hyperemesis gravidarum, or in the case administration of diuretics, in respiratory alkalosis or in cases of urinary infections by urease-producing germs such as Proteus miriabilis or in cases of a vegetarian diet [18].

In patients with alkanuria an alkaline pH is reported, which occurs in the presence of bacteria, urinary infection or diets rich in citrus or vegetables or the presence of certain drugs. It is also the product of the presence of lithiasis due to calcium carbonate, calcium phosphate and magnesium phosphate. However, the presence of acid urine is identified with aciduria, the product of respiratory or metabolic acidosis. When there is tubular acidosis, the urine is alkaline and the blood pH shows acidity [19].

During the pregnancy motivated by the MFE, changes in the breathing of the pregnant woman begin to appear from the eighth week, they begin with hyperventilation and a slight dyspnea which increases gradually throughout the pregnancy due to anatomical modifications by increasing the internal vertical diameters. and circumference of the ribcage when the uterus increases in size and volume, which in turn compresses the abdominal viscera against the diaphragm, thereby limiting its mobility, thereby increasing intra-abdominal pressure, which has its impact at the of lung volumes. This in turn causes the reduction of PCO2 to 30 mmHg by the action of progesterone, while increasing PO2 to 107 mmHg. Serum bicarbonate decreases to 20 mEq/L. By increasing renal excretion, it modifies the pH from 0.02 to 0.06 as a metabolic compensation for respiratory alkalosis (4.5).

All of this has as a consequence that the urine tends to become alkaline with a Ph of 6.0 or more, which, together with the gravid changes that affect the urinary system, will favor the appearance of UTI.

2.4 Hormonal study in a urine sample

Human chorionic gonatropin (HCG) is a protein synthesized by embryonic tissues, made up of 2 amino acid chains called alpha and beta. Its secretion is related to the growth of trophoblastic tissue during pregnancy, reaching its maximum levels between weeks 3 and 9 of the same [20].

Its concentration varies substantially in serum and urine [20]. For this reason, excretion in urine has allowed the development of pregnancy tests due to their levels in urine to make a diagnosis of it in a simple way, which can be carried out by patients without the need to go to a laboratory, but without specifying the conditions. Weeks of gestation, which is done by evaluating the plasmatic levels of its beta fraction.

It is considered responsible for the nausea and vomiting of pregnancy. Its presence, in addition to allowing the diagnosis of normal pregnancy, allows the diagnosis of ectopic pregnancy or gestational trophoblastic disease in any of its forms, which in most cases can occur with hypertensive disorders of pregnancy when its levels quadruple the values of the normal pregnancies. However, it can give false negatives when performed between weeks 41 and 109 of pregnancy, due to the decrease in trophoblastic tissue that produces it [20].

2.5 Presence of metabolites in urine

2.5.1 Ketone bodies

The presence of ketone bodies in urine during EMB may be related to the presence of diabetes mellitus. It must be known if this diabetes was type I or II and was present before it or if it is gestational diabetes that develops during it from the 24th week of pregnancy and which can disappear after it or the patient remains diabetic. Type II [21].

The MFE that leads to changes in energy distribution during pregnancy must be taken into account [21]. At the beginning of EMB, there is an increase in insulin sensitivity with a decrease in fasting plasma glucose levels and a slight decrease in hepatic glucose production. At the end of the first trimester and during the second trimester of gestation, insulin sensitivity decreases, finding its highest level in the third trimester, with a 30% increase in hepatic glucose secretion and a 40–50% decrease in glucose mediated by insulin, leading to decreased insulin sensitivity with a predisposition to accelerated fasting ketosis and increased fasting maternal glycemia and fatty acids [21].

Gestational diabetes is a common disorder that can affect pregnancy, capable of causing maternal and fetal complications such as neural tube malformations that include anencephaly, spina bifida, renal agenesis and hypoplasia, cardiac disorders such as tetralogy of Fallot, atrioventricular septal defects., coarctation of the aorta, ventricular septal defect, and musculoskeletal diseases and injuries such as agenesis of the sacrum, cleft palate, and high risk of preeclampsia, preterm delivery, fetal malformations, and cesarean sections due to the presence of fetal macrosomia [21–23].

Diabetic ketoacidosis in gestational diabetes has an incidence of 0.3 to 5%, so it is always necessary to rule out a history of type I and II diabetes, which are more easily and severely complicated than in non-pregnant patients [24].

2.5.2 Proteinuria

A separate chapter is constituted by proteinuria in pregnancy, which is extremely important for the diagnosis, evaluation, and prognosis of hypertensive disorders of pregnancy, preeclampsia-eclampsia, and its complications. It occurs in 2 to 10% of pregnancies [25] and is responsible for 26% of maternal deaths in Latin America and 9% in Africa and Asia.

Preeclampsia affects the endothelium systemically, proving a generalized endotheliosis that reaches all organs of the economy. In the kidney, at the level of the renal glomerulus, it produces glomeruloendotheliosis, which is manifested by proteinuria and oliguria that improves after fetal extraction [25].

It is necessary and important to know the classification of hypertensive disorders of pregnancy:

1. Chronic arterial hypertension: that which occurs before 20 weeks of gestation. It may or may not have been previously diagnosed [26].

2. Gestational hypertension: It occurs after the 20th week of gestation with the absence of proteinuria and without biochemical or hematological alterations and without repercussions on fetal growth [26].

3. White coat hypertension: It appears during the visit of the patients to be checked by their doctor either in the hospital or clinic where it can reach 140/90 mmHg and when they get home it returns to levels of 120/70 mmHg [26].

4. Transient gestational hypertension: Hypertension that appears from the 2nd trimester of pregnancy, without proteinuria, which normalizes after several repeated doses at rest without persistence in the puerperium [26].

5. Pre-Eclampsia: Hypertension diagnosed after 20 weeks of gestation accompanied by proteinuria with or without renal damage, liver dysfunction, neurological abnormalities, hemolysis, thrombocytopenia and fetal growth restriction [26].

It is necessary to consider the presence of renal disease prior to pregnancy, which can cause proteinuria, for which it is necessary that it be present before the 20th week of gestation [27]. Its appearance after week 20 may constitute one of the first signs of the appearance of hypertensive disorders of pregnancy: preeclampsia [26].

For the diagnosis of proteinuria it is necessary to collect 24-hour urine with values equal to or greater than 300 mg/day [26].

In the presence of proteinuria, it is necessary to rule out different nephropathies ranging from chronic kidney disease in which a progression of kidney disease is considered [28], diabetes mellitus, human immunodeficiency virus (HIV) infection or autoimmune diseases such as Lupus. systemic erythematosus [29]. For this reason, any proteinuria greater than 300 mg/day needs to be evaluated and the respective differential diagnoses made, especially in the presence of autoimmune diseases.

Since preeclampsia is a cause of maternal morbidity and mortality in many countries [25], methods have been sought to simplify the diagnosis of proteinuria in pregnancy. One of the simplest is using Robert's reagent which produces protein precipitation forming a clear halo in a test tube which contains a urine sample. Densitometers have also been used to measure the increase in urinary density due to the increase in the proteins present in them. Its biggest disadvantage is that it can produce false positives, in which case it is necessary to resort to other tests to verify its results.

At present, test strips are used for a quick and simple diagnosis of proteinuria, easy to handle and apply both by primary health personnel in a prenatal consultation, and for use by the patient at home [30]. Although they can give results as false positives or negatives, motivated by the fact that the presence of pathologies prior to pregnancy or not must be known, it is useful in patients with blood pressures of 140/90 mmHg, for monitoring at home, which allows go to a care center if they are positive [30].

Another method that has been used to diagnose proteinuria in hypertensive disorders of pregnancy is the use of sulfosalicylic acid, looking for a fast, simple, economical and reproducible method for health personnel at any level. This chemical reagent is capable of producing protein precipitation through urine acidification. It has a sensitivity of 41.1% and a specificity of 97.7% [27].

Gestational proteinuria has been described in the absence of hypertensive disorders of pregnancy, which appears after 20 weeks of pregnancy. A careful evaluation of the same is necessary [31] motivated by the fact that previous pathologies must be ruled out, and take into account that it may be an early sign of preeclampsia [32].

Investigators have been looking for another method for the diagnosis of preeclampsia through urinalysis, which is why the presence of podocytes in urine or podocyturia has been described [33]. The podocyte is a cell that forms part of the basal epithelium of the glomerulus which is affected by renal pathologies, but it was thought that it was not altered in preeclampsia, but when the glomeruloendotheliosis of preeclampsia develops, these are affected. For this reason, the study of podocyturia as a diagnostic method for preeclampsia has been proposed. However, it is also present in cases of chronic arterial hypertension, diabetes mellitus and gestational diabetes, lupus nephritis, and chronic membranous nephropathy [30, 33]. For its study, synaptopodin is used as a marker, which is a protein that binds the actin of the podocytes with the cytoskeleton of the cells [33, 34].

2.5.3 Other analyzable metabolites in urine samples

Another method used for the diagnosis, evolution and prognosis of hypertensive disorders of pregnancy is the creatinine protein index. It is used as a simpler and faster option to perform proteinuria in 24 hours. It has a sensitivity of 90% and a specificity of 80% [35, 36].

Studies are underway to develop other methods for examining urine samples and using nuclear magnetic resonance techniques to diagnose the presence of specific metabolites or biomarkers for diagnosis of preeclampsia, gestational diabetes, preterm labor, and trisomy 21 [37].

With the appearance of the omics revolution, where through the analysis of metabolites and proteins of DNA and RNA in order to carry out diagnoses and treatments of different pathologies. These metabolomics search for low molecular weight cellular compounds such as carbohydrates, amino acids, peptides, nucleic acids, organic acids, vitamins, and lipids. They can be detected using nuclear magnetic resonance spectrometry methods in samples of blood, urine, amniotic fluid, tissue secretions, and placental tissue. These data are evaluated through computer programs where they are analyzed, studied to give their interpretation and use these data in prevention, evolution, treatment and prognosis.

These studies can be carried out at the prenatal level, during the control itself, and they can be carried out through a urine sample [38].

Diaz et al. [39] in urine samples from the 14th week of pregnancy, searched for metabolic signatures using nuclear magnetic resonance metabolomin, which revealed specific urinary metabolic signatures for malformations of the central nervous system, trisomy 21, preterm delivery, diabetes pregnancy, intrauterine growth restriction and preeclampsia, demonstrating the value of the urinalysis profile as a complementary method of diagnosis and early prediction of various disorders that occur during pregnancy [39].

Cantowine et al. [40] found urinary concentrations of Bisphenaol A and Phosphate, a metabolite which are man-made products for industrial use in a wide variety of products ranging from the lining of canned food containers, water bottles and pipes water supply, products that are released in an innocuous way to the general population throughout the world, the general population being exposed to them.

It has been shown that BFA can affect the proliferative process of trophoblast cells through an estrogen receptor with an effect of apoptosis of trophoblast cells through tumor necrosis factors which act on the placenta and therefore on the development of preeclampsia [40].

Taking into account that preeclampsia occurs more frequently in primiparous women, the use of Fit-1 tyrosine kinase has been proposed, which constitutes a promising biomarker for preeclampsia obtained from a urine sample. It is a growth factor antagonist and vasoconstrictor and sensitizes the endothelium to respond to stress and endothelial dysfunction. The study is performed with nuclear magnetic resonance spectrophotometry. The Fit-1 measures moderate to severe placental dysfunction, knowing that the development of preeclampsia occurs due to inadequate placentation with abnormal development of placental vessels at the time of trophoblastic invasion, creating high-resistance vessels instead of low-resistance ones. Resistance that occurs in normal pregnancies. For this reason, it is capable of measuring the development of preeclampsia [41].

Other metabolites and biomarkers developed from a urine sample include increased excretion of amino acids as a result of kidney damage from preeclampsia. Choline increases in these patients while glycine decreases at the same time [42].

3. Conclusions

The physiological modifications of the pregnancy through its adaptive changes, favor the development of the pregnancy, keep the expectant mother in balance to achieve its completion with the best results. However, in turn they can contribute to the appearance of pathologies caused by the lack of adaptation or poor adaptation to it, such as hypertensive disorders of pregnancy, gestational diabetes, or UTI, among others. In the effort to prevent, diagnose, treat and have an adequate prognosis, it is sought to be able to make simple and reliable diagnoses and the evaluation of uranalysis is one of the simplest methods that we have. The sample is easy to obtain and its analysis ranges from the use of reactive tapes to the diagnosis of glycosuria, proteinuria or a UTI. Urinary sediment and Ph allow us complementary diagnoses that make us suspect other pathologies such as pyelonephritis, gallbladder and renal lithiasis, facilitating their diagnosis. We must always clinically evaluate the patient according to the signs and symptoms they present in order to make the most assertive diagnosis possible. The presence of proteinuria should always make us suspect a hypertensive disorder of pregnancy, although its absence does not thus rule it out from the presence of renal pathologies or other systemic diseases present before pregnancy. The development of new techniques for evaluating a urine sample are the next stage in the diagnosis of pathologies through the metabolites excreted in the urine, which include the diagnosis of chromosomopathies, for which the urine test in pregnancy reaches every ever-greater importance.

Conflict of interest

"The authors declare no conflict of interest."

Author details

Noren Villalobos[1,2]

1 High Risk Obstetric Service, Department of Obstetrics and Gynecology, University Hospital of Maracaibo, Dr. Armando Castillo Plaza Maternity, Maracaibo, Venezuela

2 Medicine School, School of Medicine, University of Zulia, Maracaibo, Venezuela

*Address all correspondence to: norenvi@hotmail.com

References

[1] Tejada Pérez P, Cohen A, Font Arreaza IJ, Bermúdez C, Schuitemaker Requena JB. Modificaciones fisiológicas del embarazo e implicaciones farmacológicas: maternas, fetales y neonatales. Revista de Obstetricia y Ginecología de Venezuela. 2007;**67**(4):246-267

[2] Carrillo-Mora P, García-Franco A, Soto-Lara M, et al. Cambios fisiológicos durante el embarazo normal. Revista de la Facultad de Medicina de la UNAM. 2021;**64**(1):39-48. DOI: 10.22201/fm.24484865e.2021.64.1.07

[3] Vinturache A, Khalil A, GLob. Maternal physiological changes in pregnancy in the continuous textbook, women's medicine series – obstetrics module. In: Khalil A, editor. Vol. 4. London: GLOWM; 2021. pp. 1-39

[4] Vinturache A, Khalil A, Global Library of Women's Medicine. DOI: 10.3843/glown.411323

[5] Purizaca M. Modificaciones fisiológicas en el embarazo. Rev Per Ginecol Obstet. 2010;**56**:57-69

[6] Carlin A, Alfirevic Z. Physiological changes of pregnancy and monitoring. Best Practice & Research Clinical Obstetrics and Gynaecology. 2008;**22**(5):801-823

[7] Ruiz-Rodríguez M, Sánchez-Martínez Y, Suárez Cadena FC, García Ramírez JC. Prevalence and characterization of urinary tract infection in socially vulnerable pregnant women in Bucaramanga. Colombia. 2019;**69**(2):1-10. DOI: 10.15446/revfacmed

[8] Mattuizzi A, Madar H, Froeliger A, Brun S, Sarrau M, Bardy C, et al. Infección urinaria y embarazo. EMC – Ginecología-Obstetricia. 2018;**54**(4):1-20

[9] Myers VC, Muntwiler E, Bill AH. The acid-base balance disturbance of pregnancy. The journal of biological chemestry. 1931;**98**(1):253-260

[10] Platte RO, Kim ED. Urinary Tract Infections in Pregnancy. Available from: https://emedicine.medscape.com/article/452604-overview

[11] Werter DE, Kazemier BM, van Leeuwen E, et al. Diagnostic work-up of urinary tract infections in pregnancy: Study protocol of a prospective cohort study. BMJ Open. 2022;**12**:e063813. DOI: 10.1136/bmjopen-2022-063813

[12] Faneite P, Pérez Alonso MM, Sánchez WJ. In: González F, editor. Epidemiología y factores etiológicos. En Manejo del Parto Pretérmino. Caracas: Sociedad Venezolana de Obstetricia y Ginecología; 2012

[13] Fogazzi GB. The Urinary Sediment. An Integrated View. Third ed. Milano: Editorial Elsevier Srl; 2010. p. 251

[14] Ho ML, Liu WF, Tseng HY, Yu-Tzu Yeh YT, Tseng WT, et al. Quantitative determination of leukocyte esterase with a paper-based device. RSC Advances. 2020;**10**:27042. DOI: 10.1039/d0ra03306e

[15] Pfaller MA, Koontz FP. Laboratory evaluation of leukocyte esterase and nitrite tests for the detection of bacteriuria. Journal of clinical microbiology. 1985;**21**(5):840-842

[16] Estrada-Altamirano A, Figueroa-Damián R, Villagrana-Zesati R. Infección de vías urinarias en la mujer

embarazada. Importancia del escrutinio de bacteriuria asintomática durante la gestación. Perinatol Reprod Hum. 2010;**24**(3):182-186

[17] Myriam Ruiz-Rodríguez M, Sánchez-Martínez Y, Suárez-Cadena FC, García-Ramírez JC. Prevalence and characterization of urinary tract infection in socially vulnerable pregnant women in Bucaramanga, Colombia. Rev. Fac. Med. 2021;**69**(2):e77949. DOI: 10.15446/revfacmed.v69n2.77949

[18] Pagana K, Pagana T. Indicaciones e interpretación de resultados. In: Laboratorio Clínico. Primera edición en español ed. México: Editorial Manual moderno; 2014

[19] Prieto Valbuena JM, Yuste Ara JR. La clínica y el laboratorio. 23 edición ed. Barcelona: Elsevier editores; 2019. pp. 1160

[20] Velázquez N. La hormona gonadotrofina coriónica humana. Una molécula ubícua y versátil. Parte I. Rev Obstet Ginecol Venez. 2014;**74**(2):122-133

[21] Brajkovich I, Febres Balestrini F, Camejo M, Palacios A. Manual Venezolano De Diabetes Gestacional. Rev Venez Endocrinol Metab. 2016;**14**(1):56-90

[22] McMicking J, Lam AYR, et al, Global Library of women's Medicine, DOI: 10.3843/GLOWM.416413

[23] Vigil-De Gracia P, Olmedo J. Diabetes gestacional: conceptos actuales. Ginecología y Obstetricia de México. 2017;**85**(6):380-390

[24] Guevara-Valerio H, Mari-Zapata DD, Arévalo-Villa DI, Vargas-Aguilar DM, Etulain-González JE. Cetoacidosis diabética durante el embarazo: reporte de un caso. Ginecología y Obstetricia de México. 2020;**88**(7):471-476. DOI: 10.24245/gom. V88i7.3547

[25] Pérez M, Pacheco M, Pérez K, Tineo N. Daño renal en pacientes preeclámpticas con criterios de gravedad. Revista de Obstetricia y Ginecología de Venezuela. 2020;**80**(3):176-186

[26] Kane SC, Wium L, et al, Global Library of women's Medicine. DOI: 10.3843/GLOWM.413253

[27] Velásquez Penagos JA, Zuleta Tobón JJ, López Jaramillo JD, Gómez Marulanda NL, Gómez Gallego J. Use of sulfosalicylic acid in the detection of proteinuria and its application to hypertensive problems in pregnancy. Iatreia. 2011;**24**(3):259-265

[28] Cravedi P, Remuzzi G. Pathophysiology of proteinuria and its value as an outcome measure in chronic kidney disease. British Journal of Clinical Pharmacology. 2013;**76**(4):516-523. DOI: 10.1111/bcp.12104

[29] Blom K, Odutayo A, Bramham K, Hladunewich MA. Pregnancy and glomerular disease a systematic review of the literature with management guidelines. Clinical Journal of the American Society of Nephrology. 2017;**12**:1862-1872. DOI: 10.2215/CJN.00130117

[30] Jakubowski BE, Stevens R, Wilson H, Lavallee L, Brittain L, Crawford C, et al. Cross-sectional diagnostic accuracy study of self-testing for proteinuria during hypertensive pregnancies: The UDIP study. BJOG: An International Journal of Obstetrics and Gynaecology. 2022;**129**(13):2142-2148. DOI: 10.1111/1471-0528.17180

[31] Kattah A, Milic N, White W, Garovic V. Spot urine protein measurements in normotensive

pregnancies, pregnancies with isolated proteinuria and preeclampsia. American Journal of Physiology. Regulatory, Integrative and Comparative Physiology. 2017;**313**:R418-R424. DOI: 10.1152/ajpregu.00508.2016

[32] Morikawa M, Mayama M, Noshiro K, Saito Y, Nakagawa Akabane K, Umazume T, et al. Earlier onset of proteinuria or hypertension is a predictor of progression from gestational hypertension or gestational proteinuria to preeclampsia. Scientific Reports. 2021;**11**:12708. DOI: 10.1038/s41598-021-92189-w

[33] Jim B, Jean-Louis P, Qipo A, Garry DA, Mian S, Matos T, et al. Podocyturia as a diagnostic marker for preeclampsia amongst high-risk pregnant patients. Journal of Pregnancy. 2012;**2012**:984630. DOI: 10.1155/2012/984630

[34] Ning L, Suleiman HY, Miner JH. Synaptopodin is dispensable for Normal Podocyte homeostasis but is protective in the context of acute Podocyte injury. JASN. 2020;**31**:2815-2832. DOI: 10.1681/ASN.2020050572

[35] Díaz Colina NG, Chiroque Parra IR, García J, Villalobos Inciarte NE. Estudio comparativo entre la índice proteína/creatinina en una muestra de orina al azar y proteinuria en 24 horas como método diagnóstico de preeclampsia. Revista de Obstetricia y Ginecología de Venezuela. 2022;**82**(1):59-66. DOI: 10.51288/00820108

[36] Pérez Dubuc KV, Vargas Torres PA, Gil Villegas Y, Vásquez Paredes LC. Trastornos hipertensivos del embarazo: relación del índice proteína/creatinina en orina esporádica y proteinuria en 24 horas. Revista de Obstetricia y Ginecología de Venezuela. 2022;**82**(3):297-308. DOI: 10.51288/00820305

[37] Mayrink J, Leite DF, Nobrega GM, et al. Prediction of pregnancy-related hypertensive disorders using metabolomics: A systematic review. BMJ Open. 2022;**12**:e054697. DOI: 10.1136/bmjopen-2021-054697

[38] Monni G, Atzori L, Corda V, Dessolis F, Iuculano A, Hurt KJ, et al. Metabolomics in prenatal medicine: A review. Frontiers in Medicine. 2021;**8**:645118. DOI: 10.3389/fmed.2021.645118

[39] Diaz SO, Barros AS, Goodfellow BJ, et al. Second trimester maternal urine for the diagnosis of trisomy 21 and prediction of poor pregnancy outcomes. Journal of Proteome Research. 2013;**12**(6):2946-2957. DOI: 10.1021/pr4002355

[40] Cantonwine DE, Meeker JD, Ferguson KK, Mukherjee B, Hauser R, McElrath TF. Urinary concentrations of Bisphenol a and phthalate metabolites measured during pregnancy and risk of preeclampsia. Environmental Health Perspectives. 2016;**124**(10):1651-1655. DOI: 10.1289/EHP188

[41] Austdal M, Skråstad RB, Gundersen AS, Austgulen R, Iversen A-C, et al. Metabolomic biomarkers in serum and urine in women with preeclampsia. PLoS One. 2014;**9**(3):e91923. DOI: 10.1371/journal.pone.0091923

[42] Austdal M, Brettas Silva G, Bowe S, Vestrheim Thomsen LC, Haugstad Tangerås L, Bjørge L, et al. Metabolomics identifies placental dysfunction and confirms Flt-1 (FMS-like tyrosine kinase receptor 1) biomarker specificity. Hypertension. 2019;**74**:1136-1143. DOI: 10.1161/HYPERTENSIONAHA.119.13184